Ophthalmology in Medicine:
An Illustrated Clinical Guide

PRACTICAL PROBLEMS IN MEDICINE

Ophthalmology in Medicine:
An Illustrated Clinical Guide

David Abrams, DM, FRCS

Consultant Ophthalmic Surgeon, Royal Free Hospital, London

MARTIN DUNITZ

First published in the United Kingdom in 1990
by Martin Dunitz Ltd, 154 Camden High Street, London NW1 ONE

British Library Cataloguing in Publication Data

Abrams, J.D.
   Ophthalmology in medicine
   I. Ophthalmology
   1. Title
   617.7

   ISBN 0-948269-42-1

Phototypeset by Scribe Design, Gillingham, Kent
Printed and bound in Singapore by Times Offset Pte. Ltd.

To Anita — who thought I was playing bridge

Contents

Preface

This book is intentionally designed for easy and quick reference to those eye conditions that are frequently met, the way they usually present and how they are managed. As a compact overview of the subject, it should be useful to general medical practitioners and specialists in other fields of medicine, to medical students and to those in the optical profession both qualified and in training who do not wish to get bogged down in the minutiae of an enormous tome on eye disease.

The book is divided into three parts, all of which are related but have differing aims.

- Part 1 is orientated towards diagnosis of eye conditions by the non-specialist. It lays emphasis on the significance of the history of the complaint, supplemented by an appropriate but necessarily limited examination. Some of the commoner eye conditions are enumerated in relation to the symptoms and signs described, but fuller accounts of these are found in Parts 2 and 3.
- Part 2 aims to give basic formal descriptions of the main conditions. Each of the conditions is grouped as (1) a disturbance of the visual apparatus (2) an anomaly of the protective mechanism or (3) some kind of incoordination of the two eyes. Where appropriate, the routine and specialist examinations performed by the ophthalmologist are described.
- Part 3 discusses matters of general ophthalmology both from within the subject itself and in relation to other disciplines. These chapters emphasize the frequently overlapping topics of common interest to the ophthalmologist and the specialist concerned. There has been some judicious pruning of specialties as it is arguable that an interrelationship can be found between ophthalmology and practically every other speciality.

Cross reference between the three sections is inevitable, but to a certain extent they can be read independently:
- Part 1 as a diagnostic *vade mecum*
- Part 2 as a mini textbook of ophthalmology
- Part 3 as a guide to the place of ophthalmology in the general medical scheme of things.

This independence between the parts has been further encouraged by some duplication of the material.

Emphasis throughout the book is on the commonly occurring conditions; the word 'rarely' is rarely found. The reader should refer to larger texts (indicated in the Select Bibliography) if some unusual topic is not mentioned, or if the elaboration of a topic appears incomplete. In particular, those details of anatomy and pathology not having established clinical relevance, however intrinsically important, have been intentionally omitted.

It is assumed that the reader has some elementary knowledge of the structure and optics of the eye, acquired in general and pre-clinical studies. This book is therefore essentially a basic clinical presentation of the subject.

Acknowledgments

It is a pleasure to acknowledge my great debt to colleagues who have supplied me with illustrations. These include Professor Neil McIntyre, Professor Wallace Foulds, Tony Chignell, Binnie Dandona, Andrew Dhillon, Bob Dick, Bill Dinning, Ian Mackie, Marie Restori, Imri Sarkany and Alan Valentine.

I am particularly indebted to the staff of the Royal Free Hospital, notably my colleagues, Clare Davey and John Bolger, as well as to the Medical Illustration Unit of the Royal Free Hospital School of Medicine, who have been so helpful. My thanks, too, to Peter Harvey for casting a critical eye over the section on neurology.

My own secretary, Bunny Morgan, and editors Mary Banks and Pat Knightley, deserve special mention for their tireless efforts and seemingly infinite patience.

D. A.

PART 1: THE PRESENTATION OF COMMON EYE DISEASES

The complaints of patients regarding vision or some abnormality of the eye itself, or of its surrounding structures, form the bulk of this part of the book. As far as examination techniques are concerned, a comparison is made between those appropriate to the non-specialist and those carried out by the ophthalmologist or optician. In order to make this comparison, a clarification of the roles of the various professionals concerned with eye disease is first given.

It is hoped that, using this information, the non-specialist will pay great attention to the patient's history, will be conscious of the limitations of his examination techniques and, finally, will make the right decisions on referral.

1   Normal sight and how it may fail

Central to the whole subject of eye disease is the patient's complaint of a deterioration in the sight of one or both eyes. To appreciate the ways in which a patient's vision can be affected, it is helpful to understand the mechanism of normal vision.

NORMAL VISION

The structures of the eyeball (the camera of the visual system) are coordinated so that, in normal vision, rays of light from a distant viewed object pass through optically transparent elements. These are, the cornea, aqueous humour, lens and vitreous humour (Figure 1.1). The elements focus the rays sharply as an inverted image on a light-sensitive layer, the retina. By an alteration in the shape of the lens (the process known as accommodation), the retinal image can be kept sharp when an object occupies a position requiring near vision (Figure 1.2).

The retina lines a large part of the back of the eyeball, but a particular part of it, the central area known as the macula, is responsible for the most refined vision; it is on to this area that any object requiring special attention is imaged. The macula therefore subserves central vision.

The retina consists of many layers of nerve cells and fibres, but the actual light-sensitive cells are of two types, cones and rods (Figure 1.3).

● Cones are responsible for day vision, for the accurate perception of forms and shapes, and for colour vision; they predominate in the macular area, although they are present elsewhere in the retina.

● Rods come into play for night vision and are widely distributed throughout the retina, though they are scarce at the macula itself.

The rods and cones are situated in a layer on the outer aspect of the retina, and light has to pass through the inner retinal layers in order to reach them.

Nervous impulses from the rods and cones are transmitted via various cells and fibres of the retina, eventually to pass out of the eyeball into the optic nerve and the visual pathway. Finally they reach the visual part of the cerebral cortex at its most posterior part, the occipital lobe. The signals from the two eyes are processed (analogous, one might say, to the developing and printing of a photographic system) so that a single erect image is received in consciousness.

Clear sight therefore depends on three essential components:

1 A sharply focused retinal image

2 The functional integrity of the retina

3 An intact visual pathway and visual cortex.

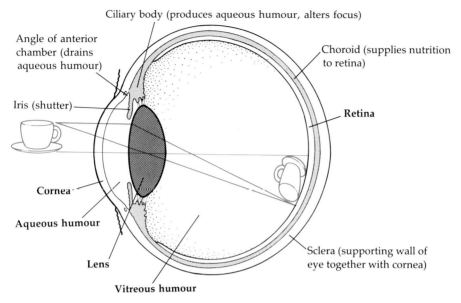

Ciliary body (produces aqueous humour, alters focus)

Angle of anterior
chamber (drains
aqueous humour)

Choroid (supplies nutrition
to retina)

Iris (shutter)

Retina

Cornea

Aqueous humour

Sclera (supporting wall of
eye together with cornea)

Lens

Vitreous humour

Figure 1.1   The structures of the eyeball. Those
directly concerned with vision are labelled in bold type.

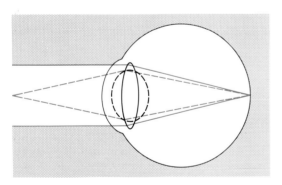

Figure 1.2   Accommodation. The lens bulges,
increasing its optical converging power.

If any of these essential components is lacking,
the vision will to some degree be defective.

BLURRED VISION

It is always possible to explain blurred vision on
the basis of the three components mentioned

above. In other words, the cause will be a poor
quality retinal image, some disease of the retina
itself, or a neuro-ophthalmic disorder.

Defects of the retinal image

The conditions degrading the retinal image may
be subdivided into two categories: optical causes
and opacities of the ocular media.

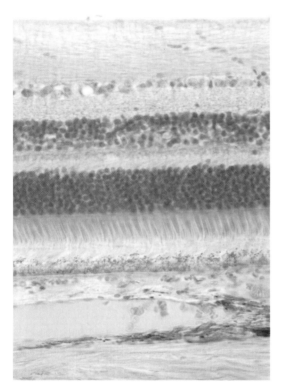

Figure 1.3 A photomicrograph of the retina, choroid and sclera. The broad dense layer is that of the nuclei of the rods and cones. The cones are immediately next to the pigment epithelium, separated here by an artefactual gap. The inner aspect of the retina is above the rods and cones. It should be noted that the light has to pass through most of the layers of the retina before reaching the rods and cones.

Optical causes In practice an unclear retinal image is the commonest cause of the complaint of blurred vision and is most likely to be due to an optical disturbance—one of the refractive errors, for example, myopia, hypermetropia, presbyopia or astigmatism (see Chapter 7). In these conditions, no actual disease of the eyeball is present, but refraction does not form a clear image on the retina. It is as if the 'camera' is simply not focused properly.

1 Blurred distance vision is the characteristic of myopia (short-sightedness)

2 Blurred near vision may occur in hypermetropia (long-sightedness)

3 Blurred near vision is also the presenting complaint of presbyopia, owing to progressive loss of the power of accommodation. As noted, this is a function leading to increased curvature of the surfaces of the lens of the eye, allowing it to change focus from far to near distances. Presbyopia typically starts in middle age.

It is important to realize that while refractive errors are the commonest conditions giving rise to blurred vision, they never cause severe loss of sight, neither do they occur acutely. An optometrist or optician is professionally trained to recognize and treat such optical errors with spectacles or contact lenses.

Opacities of the ocular media The refractive errors apart, an important group of conditions that cause blurred vision are the opacities of the normally clear ocular media.

The media (the cornea, aqueous humour, lens and vitreous) can become cloudy at any time of life, but the commonest and most important condition is senile cataract (see Chapter 10), an opacification occurring in the lens of the eye in old age.

Retinal disease affecting vision

Blurred vision may occur in retinal disease, particularly when the central region (the macula) is involved. When the central vision is affected, it is especially difficult to see well enough to do detailed, close work and, in the elderly, degeneration of the macula is a great problem because it will interfere with reading and writing (see Chapter 12).

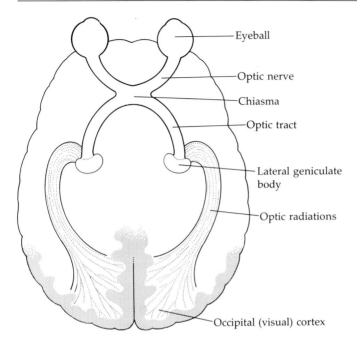

Eyeball

Optic nerve

Chiasma

Optic tract

Lateral geniculate body

Optic radiations

Occipital (visual) cortex

Figure 1.4   The visual pathway.

Retinal disease affecting parts other than the macula may be unnoticed, but if a defect of sight occurs, it takes the form of a field defect which matches up with the particular area of the retina involved. As the image on the retina is optically inverted, the patient's complaint is given in the opposite sense. For instance, if a retinal detachment occurs in, say, the nasal (medial) half of the retina, the patient will notice a 'shadow' obscuring the temporal (lateral) half of the field of vision.

Involvement of the visual pathway

Conditions involving the visual pathway (Figure 1.4) and visual cortex are numerous and the precise way in which the sight is affected depends on the whereabouts of the lesion. Disorder of one optic nerve affects the vision of the eye from which it originates. A disturbance of or behind the chiasma, where some of the optic nerve fibres from each eye cross over to the opposite side is likely to affect the field of vision of both eyes. A typical example is a homony-mous hemianopia, the loss of half the field of each eye following the common type of stroke. (This disorder is discussed more fully in Chapter 24.)

Important features of the history of visual disturbance

The important features here are as follows:

1 The severity of the disorder

2 What the onset was like

3 The course of the condition

4 Whether one or both eyes are affected

5 Whether the disturbance affects a particular visual function

6 If the sight is affected for distance and near vision, or if one of these is particularly affected

7 Particular factors making the sight worse

8 The patient's general health

9 Any family history

10 The age group of the patient.

1 *The severity of the disorder*

The severity of the disorder is the first thing to consider. While optical problems (Chapter 7) blur the sight, they never give rise to anything that the average patient would describe as losing the sight altogether, or blindness.

All other conditions affecting the sight may progress to, or indeed first appear as, a severe visual disturbance which the patient may describe as blindness.

2 *What the onset was like*

The common causes of sudden loss of vision are:

● Vascular accidents in the retina (Chapter 22) or optic nerve

● Haemorrhages into the vitreous and into the macular region of the retina (Chapters 11 and 12)

● Some cases of retinal detachment and acute glaucoma (Chapters 12 and 13)

● Optic neuritis (Chapter 24).

Although occasionally an optical problem or a cataract is noticed suddenly, it does not arise suddenly and it may simply be that the patient became aware of it at one particular juncture.

3 *The course of the condition*

If the onset of the condition was rapid, the patient's past and immediate history are important. For instance, have there been any previous episodes? Is the visual loss still present or has there been some recovery? Examples of this are subacute glaucoma (see Chapter 13) and transient ischaemic attacks (TIAs) of a much shorter duration (see Chapter 22), perhaps seconds or minutes, and migrainous interference with sight which commonly resolves after ten to twenty minutes, to be followed usually, but not invariably, by a headache (see Chapter 4).

If the disturbance was of a slow onset, is it now progressing or stationary, or is it slowly recovering as, for example after a small vitreous haemorrhage?

4 *Whether one or both eyes are affected*

Optical errors commonly affect both eyes, but not invariably. Disease of the structures of the eyeball may occur unilaterally, though the condition is often present in both eyes, perhaps to a greater extent in one than the other eye. For example, senile cataract is usually more advanced in one eye than the other.

Sudden involvement of the vision of both eyes simultaneously is most likely to arise from a cortical vascular disturbance, rarely from the eyes themselves.

5 *Whether the disturbance affects a particular visual function*

A general blur in vision should be distinguished from something involving either the central vision or a peripheral defect; a complaint, say, about the central vision only, would be most unlikely in a condition which simply interferes with the clarity of the retinal image generally.

A defect of the visual field is never an optical problem. Upper or lower (vertical) field defects are often retinal in origin. Lateral or medial defects can arise from retinal, glaucomatous or neurological conditions.

6 *If the sight is affected for distance and near vision, or if one of these is particularly affected*

Intermittent blurring of near vision is often optical in nature, arising from partial failure of accommodation which may be age-related (presbyopia) or drug-induced.

7 *Particular factors making the sight worse*

An example of other factors making the sight worse is the patient's vision being especially bad in bright light, for example, some form of cataract (see Chapter 10), or in poorly lit circumstances, such as night blindness in retinitis pigmentosa (see Chapter 12).

8 *The patient's general health*

Additional information may be obtained from the patient's general medical history. The presence of such conditions as hypertension or diabetes is obviously important in the differential diagnosis of visual disturbance.

9 *The family history*

There is sometimes a family background to major eye diseases. For instance, senile cataract may have been present in the patient's parents. Other examples of a familial and inherited tendency are high degrees of myopia and the primary glaucomas.

Another reason for enquiring about the family history is to reveal the patient's anxiety about possible causes of the deteriorating vision.

10 *The age group of the patient*

The patient's complaint may be age-related:

● Children may or may not complain about their vision, but the parents may have noticed the child peering, or a routine school examination may have found the vision to be defective. This is the period of life when refractive errors are usually first discovered, particularly myopia in the ten- to twenty-year-old age group.

● By the early twenties, most individuals needing spectacles will have been supplied with them. The next group of patients requiring spectacles will be those who were hitherto optically normal but find in their early forties that reading is progressively difficult—they have presbyopia.

● Otherwise, between the ages of twenty and fifty years, there is normally a 'quiet' period as far as visual trouble is concerned. Some hypermetropes start to need reading spectacles rather earlier than the presbyopic age group. However, from the point of view of organic disease, the most important condition in this age group is diabetes, which may give rise to retinopathy, an extremely serious affection in middle life.

● After fifty years of age, a gradual increasing incidence of cataract and primary glaucoma begin to feature (see Chapters 10 and 13). After sixty-five years of age, senile macular degeneration becomes increasingly important (see Chapter 12). Indeed, these three conditions are the main causes of defective eyesight in old age.

The age of the patient is thus a 'physical sign' which may usefully point to a likely group of conditions. The precise diagnosis, as always, depends on the appropriate findings, discussed in Chapter 6.

PRACTICAL POINTS

- Vision is defective if any of the following is lacking:
    A sharply focused retinal image
    The functional integrity of the retina
    An intact visual pathway and visual cortex.

- Blurred vision is most commonly due to one of the refractive errors.

- Other less common causes are opacities of the ocular media and retinal disease, especially at the macula.

- Detailed history-taking is an essential first step in any complaint of visual disturbance.

- The age of the patient is an important indicator of the cause.

2 Other kinds of visual disturbance

In this chapter some of the commonly occurring disturbances of sight other than visual deterioration are considered.

Distorted vision

A complaint of distortion, such as a straight line appearing to have a kink, is usually a symptom of disease of the macular region of the retina.

Double vision: diplopia

Double vision arises when, owing to a failure of coordination, the image from one eye is different from that of the other and both images are perceived simultaneously. When an incoordination occurs in a child and a squint develops, the response to the situation is for the image from one eye to be suppressed, so that binocular vision is sacrificed. Diplopia is therefore an uncommon symptom of a squint in early life. In an adult where binocular vision (seeing with both eyes) is mandatory, suppression is no longer an option and incoordination of the eyes may cause double vision.

The important clinical considerations in diplopia are:

1 Is the diplopia abolished when one or other eye is closed, that is, is the diplopia truly binocular—from the two eyes?

2 Is the diplopia worse in any particular direction?

3 Are the two images separated horizontally, vertically or both?

4 Is the diplopia constant or intermittent?

The answers to these points will give some indication, even before the examination of the ocular movements, as to which likely muscle or muscles are underacting.

Intermittent diplopia is often incorrectly taken to be symptomatic of a neurological disorder; while this may indeed be the case, far more commonly the condition arises from a latent squint, present since early life, that sometimes becomes uncontrolled.

Sudden persistent double vision in an adult is an important condition meriting not only a full ophthalmic examination, but also a general medical or neurological investigation. Many such cases never have their cause identified, and a high proportion recover spontaneously. The commonest type is a weakness of outward movement due to a VIth nerve palsy.

In all cases of diplopia, enquiry should be made to establish any history of squint in childhood (see Chapter 19), or if the patient has any general medical or neurological disorder, for example, hypertension, diabetes, dysthyroid disease or multiple sclerosis (see also Part 3).

A double or multiple image from one eye can occasionally arise in a patient with a slight degree of cataract. Furthermore, some patients may describe their vision as being double, when what they really mean is that the image is blurred.

A simple examination pertinent to diplopia and squint is described in Chapter 19.

Diplopia is a symptom which calls for referral, preferably for an ophthalmological rather than an optician's opinion, unless the term is being used to describe blurred vision, when an optician's opinion should be sought.

Floaters in the vision

A whole series of symptoms (spots, flies, spiders, cobwebs, circles, lines, hairs) may be given by the patient describing moving objects interfering with the sight. Many of these objects are due to some abnormality in the vitreous (see Chapter 11), the commonest being a simple degenerative change. The particles may be so small that they are invisible with the ophthalmoscope (so-called *muscae volitantes*).

If the degenerative process is more marked, as is particularly the case with myopic patients, objects can actually be seen in the vitreous with the ophthalmoscope.

The sudden appearance of floaters is an important symptom because it may represent an acute degenerative process, such as a posterior vitreous detachment, a small vitreous haemorrhage, or entry into the vitreous of inflammatory debris from a choroiditis or cyclitis (see Chapter 11).

Shadows in the field of vision

'Shadows' in the field of vision is sometimes simply the symptom of a vitreous opacity. On further questioning, the patient may often describe the detailed shape of the opacity.

The complaint of a shadow is also an important symptom of a defect of the visual field, which may be described by patients suffering from conditions such as a retinal detachment,

branch retinal vessel occlusion or chronic glaucoma, or it may be due to neurological causes of loss of field.

Flashes of light

The most commonly experienced flashes of light, or what are often described as such, as premonitory symptoms of migraine (see Chapter 4). The succeeding nauseous headache, the recurrent nature of the condition, and the absence of any abnormal eye signs, should assist in the diagnosis. The patient may be unable to identify whether the phenomenon is coming from one or both eyes. There may be an actual pattern or figure in a particular part of the field of vision.

A common cause of flashes, often described as electric sparks or lightning, particularly in the outer field, is posterior vitreous detachment where the flashes are often associated with floaters in the vision (see Chapter 11). These flashes are typically experienced when the patient goes from a light to a dark environment.

Flashes also occur in retinal degeneration, which may precede the formation of a hole and retinal detachment (see Chapter 12). Therefore, particularly in a highly myopic patient, flashes of light are an indication to examine the retina thoroughly, especially its periphery. In fact, any mechanical irritation of the retina may cause a sensation of flashes of light. In rare cases, this can result from a neoplasm, perhaps a malignant melanoma of the choroid.

Cerebral cortical conditions (hypertension, arteriosclerosis or tumours) may produce flashes of light, but these associations are far from common. In such cases, the flashes appear in the same part of the visual field of both eyes.

Photophobia–dazzle and glare

Patients complaining of a dislike of light, without any ocular inflammation, are commonly encountered. Their complaint is usually psychogenic, or based on an obscure desire to appear fashionable in dark glasses!

There are, however, well-recognized and genuine cases of photophobia, particularly in migraine sufferers, in some cases of general allergy (hay fever) and occasionally in meningeal irritation. Perhaps the commonest group are those patients lacking ocular pigment, ranging from the full-blown albino to the blond and fair-complexioned (see Chapter 23).

Photophobia in cases of an acute red eye virtually eliminates the diagnosis of a simple bacterial conjunctivitis and suggests iritis or corneal inflammation (see Chapter 3).

Apart from discomfort arising from exposure to light, some patients may suffer a worsening of vision in brighter rather than dimmer surroundings. This happens particularly in cases of opacities of the media which affect the main optic axis of the eye. This is because the relatively contracted pupil restricts the entering rays of light to the pathological region of the affected medium. As might be expected, eyedrops used regularly to keep the pupil permanently dilated may improve vision — for example, in cases of axial cataract.

Haloes around lights

Any patient with an unfocused retinal image may, on looking at a source of light, see a halo or halation effect around the image.

A true coloured ring with a rainbow-like effect is an important ocular symptom as it suggests the possibility of glaucoma, usually of the closed angle type (see Chapter 13). The halo is caused by oedema of the epithelium of the cornea, owing to a rise in eye pressure.

There are rarer causes of haloes around lights. For example, corneal disease may itself cause oedema, or a vaguely similar symptom is sometimes experienced by patients with early cataract.

Defective colour vision

Defective colour vision, typically a difficulty in distinguishing between red and green, is usually inherited and is much commoner in males than females.

The condition is hardly ever found to be a symptom of acquired organic eye disease, but in those occasional instances that it is, macular or optic nerve pathology is likely to be the cause.

PRACTICAL POINTS

- If any of the following symptoms is described, the non-specialist should refer the patient to an ophthalmologist

    — distorted vision
    — double vision
    — floaters or shadows in the field of vision
    — flashes of light
    — photophobia
    — haloes around lights.

3 Inflamed eyes

In considering the inflamed eye, a distinction needs to be made between an inflammation apparently of the eyeball itself and an inflammation of the surrounding tissues of the eye, particularly the eyelids. The clinical complex known as the acute red eye usually refers only to the former. Inflammation affecting the eyelids is discussed later in this chapter.

THE ACUTE RED EYE

The main causes of the acute red eye are:

- Conjunctivitis

- Corneal inflammation

- Anterior uveitis, otherwise known as iridocyclitis or iritis

- Acute glaucoma.

In these conditions, the inflammation produces an engorgement of pre-existing vessels in the conjunctiva and subconjunctival tissues. The anatomy and function of the tissues involved in ocular inflammation are illustrated in Figure 3.1.

The commonest cause of an acute red eye is acute conjuntivitis. As Figure 3.1 shows, a disturbance of the conjunctiva does not in itself produce any change in the eyeball.

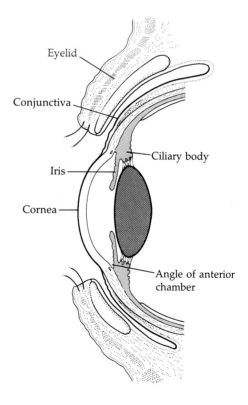

Figure 3.1 The structures concerned in the acute red eye. The posterior segment of the eyeball is intentionally omitted. Note that the conjunctiva and the eyelids are not part of the mechanism of vision and inflammation of these structures does not lead to any disturbance of the sight.

Two points of particular importance in distinguishing conjunctivitis from other causes of an acute red eye are:

1 The patient's vision

2 The state of the pupil.

In conjunctivitis, neither the patient's vision nor the pupil size or reaction is in any way abnormal. The cardinal rule for a patient with a red eye who has either blurring of the vision or some pupillary abnormality should be referral to an ophthalmologist. Such a patient should never be diagnosed or treated as having conjunctivitis.

Diagnosing the cause of an acute red eye

Differentiating the various causes of an acute red eye is, for the ophthalmologist, a relatively simple process. This is because a slit-lamp examination can be carried out (see Chapter 6), making it possible to examine minutely the anterior segment of the eye, and to measure the patient's ocular pressure.

The non-specialist does not usually have these facilities and may be unable to reach a precise diagnosis. However, by taking a short, pertinent history from the patient, followed by an examination which includes the visual acuity and the pupil, a tentative diagnosis can often be reached.

The symptoms complained of, or to be enquired for, are:

1 Simply a red eye with no other complaint

2 Stickiness or discharge; the principal symptom of conjunctivitis

3 Watering; a feature of corneal inflammation and uveitis

4 Blurred vision in the affected eye

5 Photophobia, perhaps with accompanying blepharospasm (reflex closure of the eyelids)

6 Pain; not a feature of conjunctivitis, but it may occur with the other causes of an acute red eye. Acute glaucoma in particular may give rise to severe aching pain, either in the eye itself or in the temple or forehead

7 A foreign body sensation; this may occur in conjunctivitis or in corneal ulceration.

The signs encountered, or to be looked for, are:

1 The vision of the affected eye

2 The pupil's size, its shape and reactions

3 The whereabouts of the redness (Figure 3.2). In cases of corneal inflammation and uveitis, for instance, the redness tends to be accentuated around the margin of the cornea. Localized or sectorial redness suggest episcleritis (see page 18) or mechanical irritation

4 The pressure of the eye, which can be roughly estimated without instruments (see Chapter 13)

5 Fluorescein staining of the cornea; the cardinal sign of corneal ulceration.

Conjunctivitis

A manifestly sticky eye, either complained of or possibly discovered during an examination, is an almost universal feature of bacterial conjunctivitis. If the patient does not admit to having a sticky eye, it is pertinent to ask whether the eyelids were stuck together on waking in the morning (another sign of discharge).

As noted, pain is not a feature of conjunctivitis, but the patient may experience a sandy, gritty or occasionally itchy sensation in the affected eye. Itching is a particular symptom of allergic conjunctivitis.

Corneal inflammation

Corneal inflammation occurs typically as a corneal ulcer. The condition may be painful; the pain being often described as sharp as of a foreign body, or rather aching in character. There

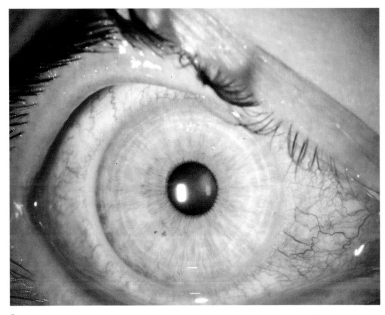

a

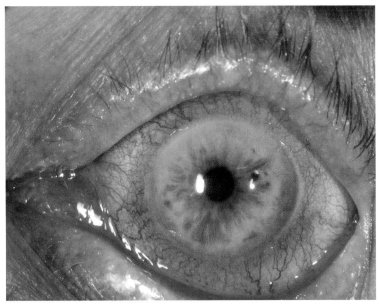

b

Figure 3.2 (*a*) Conjunctivitis: the redness of the eye is
diffuse. (*b*) In iritis (here) and also in corneal
inflammation, the redness is concentrated around the
edge of the cornea – circumcorneal injection.

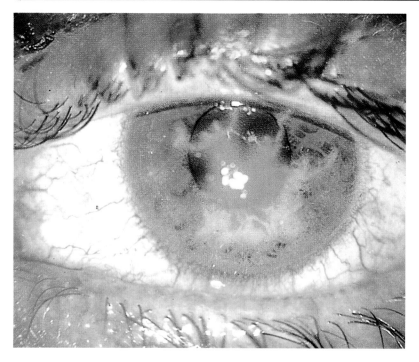

Figure 3.3 Fluorescein staining of the cornea.

may be localized redness near the site of the inflammation, and the vision is affected if the central area of the cornea opposite the pupil is involved.

Even if the central area of the cornea is not involved, vision may be disturbed by photophobia and watering. The pupil tends to be equal to, or smaller than, that of the fellow eye. The characteristic feature of a corneal ulcer is staining with the dye fluorescein (Figure 3.3).

Anterior uveitis

Commonly known as 'iritis', or iridocyclitis, the condition is characterized by a relatively small pupil (Figure 3.4) which may be irregular. Even

if the pupil is not obviously small, it may not dilate well when the eyes are covered to exclude room light.

The redness of the eye tends to be around the cornea. Additionally, photophobia is frequent and the vision is usually blurred, sometimes severely so, though occasionally the vision is normal. Aching pain in or near the eye may also be experienced.

Acute glaucoma

Acute glaucoma should always be suspected in any patient complaining of a severely painful red eye.

A marked rise in ocular pressure is the

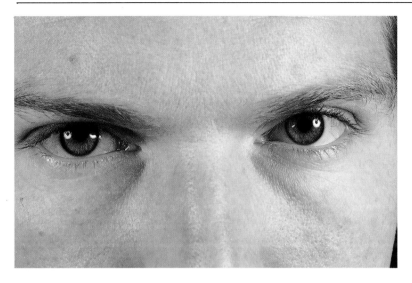

Figure 3.4   A small pupil in a case of acute red eye, suggesting, as in this case, iritis.

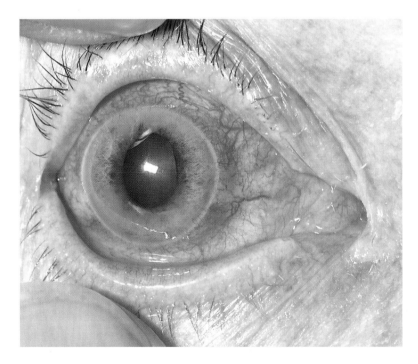

Figure 3.5   Acute glaucoma. The large pupil appears hazy because of oedema of the cornea. Note the predominantly circumcorneal injection.

principal feature of an eye with acute glaucoma (Figure 3.5). The affected eye is also palpably harder than that of the fellow eye (see Digital tonometry, Chapter 13).

Acute glaucoma can be diagnosed without reference to the ocular pressure because of other characteristic features. These are:

- A semi-dilated pupil, which does not react to light, seen through a hazy cornea

- A very painful or aching eye with blurred, or extremely poor, vision.

Other common causes of red eye

Other minor causes of a red eye are:

- Scleritis/episcleritis
- Subconjunctival haemorrhage.

Scleritis/episcleritis

Inflammation of the sclera or of the episclera (the tissue between the sclera and the conjunctiva) is a minor cause of a red eye, producing characteristically sectorial inflammation (Figure 3.6).

The condition must be distinguished from the injection resulting from a marginal corneal ulcer, which may also appear sectorial, and also from the redness produced by a mechanical irritant such as an inturning eyelash or eyelid, or by a foreign body.

Subconjunctival haemorrhage

The condition is of a slightly different nature to that of the other causes of red eye, the redness being due to blood and not to engorgement of blood vessels (see Figure 3.7).

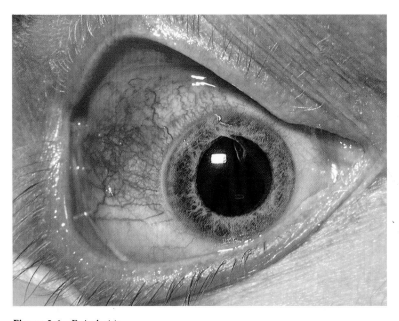

Figure 3.6 Episcleritis.

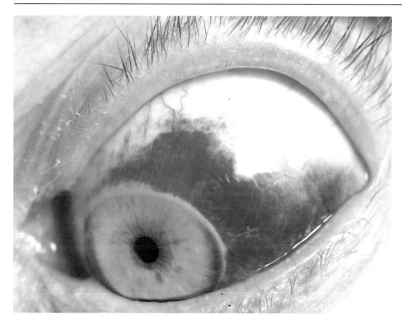

Figure 3.7 Subconjunctival haemorrhage. Note that away from the redness, the eye is completely white.

Most cases are spontaneous if there is no history of trauma and are occasionally associated with an episode of marked physical exertion. Some hypertensives and diabetics are prone to these haemorrhages. They also occur in patients with bleeding diseases and those on anticoagulants. Apart from being unsightly, there are no symptoms of a subconjunctival haemorrhage, and no treatment is necessary because the blood is normally absorbed within seven to ten days.

Referral of the acute red eye

It is advisable that the following conditions be referred for ophthalmological advice, without treatment:

● Suspected corneal inflammation usually needs to be referred because it may require frequent slit-lamp examinations to confirm the diagnosis, and to follow the effect of the treatment. If the patient's eye is not severely inflamed, simple management may lead to a rapid resolution without there being any need to refer the patient to a specialist (see Chapter 8).

● If iritis is suspected it is always best referred because again frequent slit-lamp examinations are necessary in order to make the diagnosis and to follow the course of the condition.

● Acute glaucoma. Apart from the general practitioner perhaps prescribing an analgesic, it is unwise to treat an acute red eye if acute glaucoma is suspected. This is because it is important to measure the eye pressure initially, and then to follow the pressure changes so as to assess the effectiveness of the treatment.

Any patient diagnosed initially as having conjunctivitis, but who fails to respond to simple chemotherapy within three days, should be referred for a slit-lamp examination, and possible microbiological investigation.

NEIGHBOURHOOD INFLAMMATION

Inflammation of the structures surrounding the eye, particularly the eyelids, need not necessarily be associated with redness of the eyeball itself.

An inflammation of the lid margins, blepharitis, usually involving all four eyelids may be associated with conjunctivitis (see Figure 3.8).

Inflammation of the eyelids proper occurs in two forms:

1 A generalized inflammation of the eyelids proper may show the features of an eczema—particularly if there is an allergic aetiology (see Chapter 17)

2 A localized painful inflammation of one eyelid, or nearby structure, should always prompt the search for an area of particular tenderness. This is especially so with acute infections of the lid glands, the commonest cause being a stye (Figure 3.9), an acute inflammation occurring in a lash root. An infected meibomian cyst is the next most common cause of a localized inflammation. Alternatively there may be an acute infection in part of the lacrimal apparatus either in the sac or, more rarely, in the gland itself (see Chapter 15).

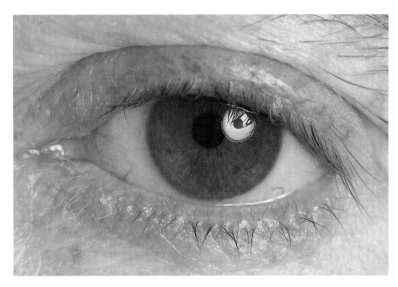

Figure 3.8 Blepharitis – inflammation of the eyelid margins.

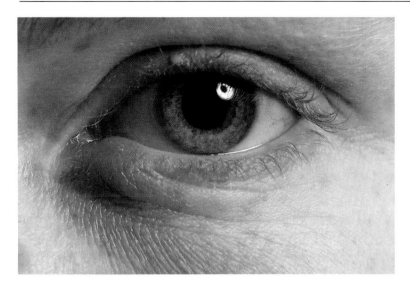

Figure 3.9   Stye.

A less common, but none the less important cause of an inflammation near to the eye is an acute inflammation of the sinuses. A particular localized form results from ethmoidal sinusitis. More widespread inflammation, orbital cellulitis, may itself be secondary to an inflammation either in the lids or in the sinuses.

The characteristic feature of the orbital cellulitis is that, in addition to the acute inflammatory swelling of the eyelids, the eyeball itself is red and protruding, proptosed, and there may be some limitation of ocular movement. In the later stages of the condition, vision may be severely affected.

In marked neighbourhood inflammations, referral is essential for an ENT opinion, either before or after appropriate radiology has been carried out.

A more localized inflammation does not usually need to be referred, as most conditions respond to local and perhaps systemic chemotherapy.

PRACTICAL POINTS

● The term 'acute red eye' refers to inflammation of the eyeball only and not the surrounding area.

● The vision, pupil size and reactions must always be assessed. If any is abnormal, the condition is not likely to be conjunctivitis.

● Conjunctivitis is typified by a sticky eye, with normal vision and a normal pupil.

● The characteristic feature of corneal ulceration is staining with fluorescein.

● A relatively small irregular pupil may indicate iritis.

● A severely painful acute red eye is likely to indicate acute glaucoma.

● For all conditions suspected of not being conjunctivitis, referral is necessary.

● Neighbourhood inflammation usually presents with lid oedema owing to infection in the lid itself, the lacrimal apparatus or sinuses.

4   Painful and uncomfortable eyes

As outlined in Chapter 3, pain may be only part of the picture of an inflamed eye. This chapter looks at the pain or discomfort arising in eyes that are not inflamed.

Eyestrain

The clinical picture of eyestrain is a group of symptoms which include the following:

- Tired, hot, dry eyes

- Sore eyelids, perhaps with excessive blinking

- Aching pain, and referred symptoms such as headache

- Intermittent blurring of vision, sometimes double vision.

These symptoms are usually found in patients who have optical errors or muscle imbalance, frequently of a mild degree.

In smaller optical errors such as early presbyopia, low degrees of hypermetropia and in astigmatism, an unusual accommodative effort may produce some improvement in sight, but the 'strain' of exercising this often gives rise to the symptoms outlined above. Where severe optical errors are present, the patient often abandons any attempt to clarify vision because the effort is not normally productive.

Similarly, if a disturbance of muscle balance (the coordination of the movement of the two eyes, to give a similar image to each one) is severe, any attempt to obtain binocular vision is usually abandoned. If the disturbance is of a lesser degree, for instance, when a strabismus is latent (heterophoria—see Chapter 19), and is prevented from showing itself by the power of binocular vision, the symptom complex of eyestrain may be experienced. The common conditions responsible are weakness of convergence, latent convergence, or intermittent divergent strabismus, which are revealed by the cover test and an examination of the ocular movements.

Even though eyestrain is often thought to be functional in the sense of psychogenic in origin, the eyes being perfectly healthy, the patient's discomfort is real enough. The functional view is perhaps supported by the fact that the symptoms of eyestrain are intensified at times of general stress or physical fatigue. Nevertheless, similar symptoms may be experienced by an absolutely normal patient performing some visual task to which he is unaccustomed, either in its degree (such as prolonged reading in poor light) or by the very nature of the task itself. A modern widespread example is the use of visual display units (VDUs), although as yet there is no conclusive evidence of any permanent harm being caused by this equipment.

It is in fact a myth that excessive use of the eyes will in some way cause damage to them; even though the symptoms of eyestrain may occur, they do not signify any irreversible pathological process.

The severity and character of discomfort varies from patient to patient, often being described as aching eyes or simply a headache. The headache of eyestrain is normally frontal or temporal in site, and may be related in time to a demanding visual task. Provided a simple examination of the eye proves negative, it is often appropriate to look for an optical cause by seeking an early referral to an optician. Persistence of the symptoms, in spite of optical correction, leaves unresolved the question of their relationship to the eye. This matter is discussed in more detail below, with particular reference to headache.

Other types of pain

Pain in or around the eye is often referred pain, rather than originating from the eye itself.

Aching pain

Aching pain may be due to high ocular pressure, glaucoma, or be referred from paranasal structures such as the paranasal sinuses or the teeth. Such pain in and above the eye is often present for a few days before the rash of ophthalmic herpes zoster appears. Migrainous neuralgia is also a possible cause. Pain around the eye, especially in the temple, may be a symptom of temporal or cranial arteritis (see below).

The type of glaucoma in which aching pain is a prominent feature is the closed angle variety (see Chapter 13), particularly the subacute attack. Occasionally, cases of acute glaucoma will present with severe pain but show little in the way of inflammation.

In chronic simple, open angle glaucoma it is very unusual for eye pressure to be raised to a level where the patient experiences pain.

If glaucoma is suspected, referral is essential. The most important examination finding is the assessment of ocular pressure, possibly digitally but certainly instrumentally and, if at all possible, while the pain is present.

Such an examination does, however, have its negative value. For instance, if the ocular pressure is normal when the pain is severe, then the pain is clearly not due to glaucoma. The symptoms associated with subacute glaucoma (misty vision and haloes around lights during an attack) should be enquired for.

Sharp pain

Sharp pain may be described as such, or be given a more precise description such as a pricking or stabbing sensation in the eye, a feeling of a foreign body or as if a piece of grit is present.

There are many possible causes for such sensations. These range from an unsuspected foreign body under the upper lid or on the cornea, to a small corneal ulcer with minimal signs of inflammation, to misdirected eyelashes either from trichiasis or because the lower lid turns inwards, entropion. Some ophthalmologists believe that the small white chalky accumulations on the inside of the eyelid, known as concretions, may also act as mechanical irritants.

In many cases, no apparent abnormality is discovered and, as with the complaints discussed above, it is not unreasonable to conclude that the condition is psychogenic in origin.

Various neuralgias

Various neuralgias, including tic, may affect the region of the eye. Of particular importance is pain above the eye in the pre-eruptive phase of herpes zoster. Even the ophthalmologist may be unable to detect any ocular or cutaneous abnormality because it is difficult to distinguish between organic or functional pain and discomfort in that region. Post-herpetic neuralgia is an unfortunate sequel to ophthalmic zoster, the eye itself being complained of as the site of a boring or burning pain.

Generally irritable eyes

A widespread complaint is of sore, burning, watering or dry eyes, symptoms found in any patient with chronic congestion of the conjunctiva, whether infective or caused by some irritant, endogenous or exogenous. Very often, however, there are no abnormal physical signs, the eyes appearing uninflamed without evidence of mechanical irritation, lacrimal drainage anomaly or poor tear production. The eye pressures are found to be normal, the eyes coordinate well and there appears to be no optical cause for the patient's discomfort. The general practitioner and ophthalmologist alike are often left simply to treat the patient with placebos such as astringents or other such time honoured remedies.

Headache and the eye

The ophthalmologist is often, and rightly, involved in the investigation of headaches for two reasons:

1 To determine whether the eyes themselves are responsible for the headache. The causes are as those described for eyestrain (see page 23), especially accommodative failure in presbyopia and convergence weakness, as well as glaucoma. The principal examination for the eyes concerns the refraction, the muscle balance and the ocular pressures.

2 To discover any ophthalmic signs indicating a general disorder, of which headache is a known symptom. The ophthalmic examination may reveal vascular changes of hypertension and the optic disc may show atrophy or papilloedema. In any event, particular neuro-ophthalmic signs should be noted. It is also especially important that examination of the visual fields is remembered, if only by confrontation (see Chapter 23).

It is uncommon for the ophthalmic examination to establish an indisputable cause for headache.

Migraine

Pain in or around the eye, or a headache unilaterally above the eye, is often due to migraine. The usual associations of the condition help to make the diagnosis. These include premonitory visual phenomena and the nausea and vomiting experienced during the time of the headache. Migraine is occasionally confused with closed angle glaucoma because pain and coloured phenomena in the vision occur in both conditions.

Traditionally migraine is considered particularly liable to occur in patients with refractive errors. Although the relationship is exaggerated, the possibility remains that, in a few instances, eyestrain does act as a psychological trigger.

Migrainous neuralgia is a particular variety of migraine giving a well-defined clinical picture of a severe frontal headache or pain in the eye. Characteristically, the condition occurs in attacks which awaken the patient from sleep and is seen most frequently in middle-aged males.

Although we are dealing here with pain and discomfort, it is important to remember that the visual disturbances of migraine, whether the shimmering, the fortification spectra or the actual loss of acuity or field, may occur without a headache following them.

Cranial arteritis

Mention should be made of cranial arteritis as a cause of often severe pain or headache in the region of the eye. Its typical situation is in the temple, hence the term 'temporal arteritis'. This is particularly important in ophthalmology because an inflammation of blood vessels may involve the arteries of the optic nerve, thus seriously affecting vision initially of one, or perhaps later, of both eyes. (This condition is discussed further in Chapter 24.)

PRACTICAL POINTS

- 'Eyestrain' is a collective term for a ocular discomfort and associated symptoms, possibly aggravated by the intense use of the eyes.

- The main causes are small refractive errors, inadequate accommodative power and muscle imbalance between the two eyes.

- Over-use of the eyes does not lead to permanent damage.

- Although painful eyes may be caused by closed angle glaucoma, this is not a common cause.

- If glaucoma is suspected, referral is essential.

- Sometimes ocular signs give a clue to general disease, of which headache is a symptom.

- An ocular cause for headaches, other than as part of eyestrain, is also uncommon.

5   Abnormal outer appearances and other complaints

This chapter looks at a miscellaneous collection of commonly occurring conditions, mostly of the external appearance of one or both eyes.

Squint or strabismus

The term 'squinting' usually means that the eyes are not looking in the same direction as each other. However, the term is sometimes used to describe eyes that are being screwed up either in an attempt by the patient to improve his blurred sight, or owing to photophobia. True squint or, to give the correct name for an ocular deviation, 'strabismus', is a frequently encountered complaint about children by their parents, though often unnoticed by children themselves; adults who have had a strabismus since childhood may present complaining of its cosmetic appearance.

Strabismus is always a matter for prompt referral for an ophthalmologist's opinion, not that of an optician. There are many reasons for this, quite apart from the fact that ultimately a surgical procedure may be necessary.

The primary investigation of a strabismus requires an authoritative, that is medical, opinion about the normality or otherwise of the patient's eyes individually. One of the objectives of treating strabismus in children is to improve the vision of the deviating eye, if defective. This is achieved by the straight eye being covered (occlusion), although such an improvement will occur only if the deviating eye is intrinsically healthy. If the eye is unhealthy, then covering the good eye will be worse than useless. It should therefore never be left to an optician or optometrist to decide if a patient is suitable for occlusion.

It is also preferable to refer cases of pseudo-strabismus, caused, for example, by a wide nose bridge, for an ophthalmologist's opinion to confirm that no true squint is present.

Other ophthalmic complaints

Other commonly presenting ophthalmic complaints are:

- Lumps and bumps around the eyes, for example, meibomian cysts, xanthelasma of the lids and pinguecula of the conjunctiva. These conditions are discussed further and illustrated in Chapters 14 and 17

- Watering eyes from blocked tear ducts or allergy

- Staring or bulging eyes, as in thyroid disease (see Chapters 16 and 25)

● Half-closed eyes, dropped eyelids, as in congenital or neurogenic ptosis; such eyes are often described incorrectly as being small. A truly small eye (microphthalmos) is very uncommon (see Chapter 17).

● Discoloured eyes, as in jaundice. This expression may occasionally be used to describe eyes of differing iris colours (heterochromia).

PRACTICAL POINTS

● All cases of strabismus should be referred promptly for an ophthalmologist's opinion.

● Other causes of complaint about the appearance of the eyes include conditions that may indicate some obvious local pathology but may also point to some general disease, as, for example, with staring eyes caused by dysthyroid conditions or discoloured eyes, as in jaundice.

6   Ophthalmic examinations: who does what?

Assessing vision and examining the eye

Every patient presenting with an ophthalmic complaint requires two types of examination; first, there is an assessment of how well or otherwise the patient can see and, second, an inspection and investigation of the eyes and other parts of the visual apparatus.

Within these two categories, there is considerable variability in the degree and thoroughness of the examination and this depends on the professional orientation of the examiner.

THE PROFESSIONALS CONCERNED WITH EYE PROBLEMS

The question of who does what in ophthalmology is sometimes puzzling. There are three groups of professionals, the last two being medically qualified:

- Opticians or optometrists
- General medical practitioners
- Ophthalmologists.

Opticians and optometrists

The terms 'optician' and 'optometrist' are interchangeable. The latter is used almost exclusively in the USA, whereas in Britain the former is more common. There are two types of opticians, ophthalmic (sight testing) or dispensing, and some practise as both.

Ophthalmic opticians Ophthalmic opticians assess the optical state of the eye (refract patients) and if they are satisfied that no other obvious abnormality is present and the vision can be adequately corrected, they will prescribe and provide spectacles or, in appropriate cases, contact lenses.

Dispensing opticians As the name suggests, they concentrate on providing spectacles to prescription. The prescriptions may be their own, if they are also ophthalmic opticians, or of either ophthalmologists or other ophthalmic opticians. Some dispensing opticians provide contact lenses.

General medical practitioners

Patients with non-visual complaints, such as a red eye or a lump on the eyelid, usually seek advice from their family practitioner. Patients with a sight defect most often go directly to an optician but some do initially consult their own doctor.

According to the doctor's perception of the problem, based upon his examination, he will decide either to manage the complaint himself or refer the patient to an optician or an ophthalmologist.

It is one of the main purposes of this book to help primary care physicians make this decision correctly.

Ophthalmologists

Ophthalmologists fall into two groups. They are both medically qualified and specialize in eye work, but are subdivided according to whether or not they carry out eye surgery.

Ophthalmic surgeons An ophthalmologist who performs eye surgery is known as an ophthalmic surgeon. This group of ophthalmologists can give the ultimate opinion on the diagnosis and management of eye disease and carry out whatever surgery is indicated.

With the exception of an emergency, a patient's initial access to the ophthalmic surgeon is usually either from an optician or through medical colleagues, such as the family practitioner or a specialist in another discipline. Whatever route is taken by the patient, a serious eye disease such as glaucoma is likely to end up in the care of an ophthalmic surgeon at a hospital or in private practice.

Non-surgical ophthalmologists The non-surgical ophthalmologist, or ophthalmic medical practitioner, belongs to an unfortunately shrinking breed, spending a significant proportion of his professional time simply in general consultative optical work. This is frequently carried out in association with dispensing opticians who make up the spectacles to his prescription. Such an ophthalmologist's examination is likely to be founded on a wider clinical experience than that of a sight-testing optician or optometrist.

THE TYPES OF EYE EXAMINATION

We are now in a position to ascribe to these various eye professionals the different emphases of their examinations.

Examination by the family practitioner or other non-specialist This will be a *simple assessment of vision* together with a short examination of the front of the eye and an inspection of the central area of the retina with an ophthalmoscope. Such a non-specialist examination does not include any significant measurement of the optical state of the eye.

Examination by an optician or optometrist The principal diagnostic test of the optician is the *sight test*, a process also known as refracting the patient. This usually includes an objective investigation of the optical state of the eye followed by a subjective testing of the patient's vision with lenses based upon the objective findings.

It is important to remember that the simple assessment of vision by the non-specialist, described below, is not a complete sight test, although it is a part of it. Similarly, a sight test is far from a complete eye examination, although in the hands of the optician, it is usually associated with a short inspection both of the front of the eye and with the ophthalmoscope. These examinations by an optician are often more extensive than those carried out by general medical practitioners.

Examinations by ophthalmologists The most rigorous and extensive clinical examinations are those carried out by ophthalmologists. These include an initial simple assessment of vision and will include also a sight test, using the same techniques as those employed by the optician. Following this, there will be a detailed examination of the front of the eye by slit-lamp examination and then a thorough inspection of the fundus with the ophthalmoscope, which in appropriate cases is carried out with the pupil dilated with drops. Complete examination also involves methods of eye pressure measurement, visual field recording and assessment of the state of the muscle balance. Outlines of these techniques are given in the relevant subsequent parts of this book, and although the non-specialist need not be concerned with the details, there are simple versions of these methods that can be profitably incorporated into a very basic ophthalmic examination.

These techniques are summarized in tabular form at the end of the chapter.

The non-specialist examinations

As we have noted, the non-specialist normally carries out a simple assessment of vision together with a limited inspection of the front of the eye and the central area of the retina with the ophthalmoscope.

Simple assessment of vision

The simple assessment of vision with and without the patient's own spectacles is always part of an eye examination, whoever carries it out. Even when the complaint is not directly about the vision, it is valuable to record the standard obtained for future reference. It is also important to record the vision of the fellow eye as well as that of the eye about which there is a particular history.

Two aspects of vision are to be considered:

- Distance vision
- Near vision.

Assessing the distance vision

This is the basic measurement of visual acuity and is usually assessed by a Snellen type (Figure 6.1a). The patient sits 6 metres (or 20 feet) away and reads as far down the chart as possible, each eye being tested individually. It will be seen that the chart consists of a series of lines and the

lower the lines, the smaller the letters become and the thinner the strokes of which the letters are composed. The lines are of a conventional denomination. If a patient reads down to the fourth line, we say that the visual acuity is 6/18 in British terminology, 20/60 in American terminology or 0.3 by the European decimal means of recording vision. What 6/18 implies is that the patient sitting at 6 metres (20 feet) away is able to read what a normal person would be able to read at 18 metres (60 feet) away. Obviously the smaller the fraction indicating the patient's recorded visual acuity, the worse this actually is.

By these criteria, normal vision should be at least 6/6 (20/20 or 1.0) although most normal subjects have an unaided vision of somewhat better than this, 6/5 in British notation.

As many patients will undoubtedly have spectacles, distance vision should be assessed first without them and then wearing any distance correction they have. When patients are asked to read the chart, they should not wear spectacles used only for reading. Such glasses, given for presbyopia (see pages 53–5), may worsen distance vision. The spectacles used for the distance test should be those used for driving or watching television, or bifocals, if worn.

The vision of the worse eye should be tested first. If, however, there is no particular complaint about the vision of one eye or if the poor vision is the same in both, then the right eye should be tested first as this prevents the patient remembering the chart when the worse eye comes to be tested. The vision recorded is that of the lowest line that is read substantially correctly.

Although the non-specialist does not become involved in testing the vision with lenses, the pinhole aperture (Figure 6.2) can be helpful. If poor vision is due to an optical defect or to some incomplete opacity of one of the ocular media, a pinhole in front of the eye will improve the visual acuity.

In some cases of course, whether with or without glasses, the patient will not be able to see the top letter on the chart and the vision can simply be recorded in these cases as less than 6/60. 6/60, the top letter on the Snellen chart, is the same as 20/200 or 0.1 m in other terminologies,

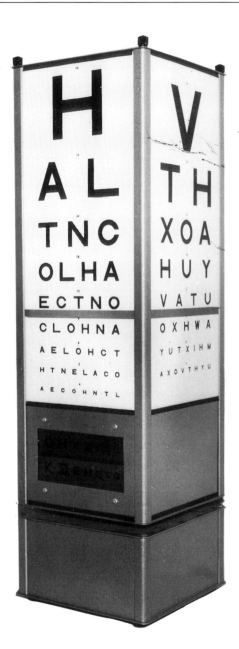

TEST-TYPES.

N.5

But the accident that followed, though it be a trifle, will be very diverting in its place. I was exceedingly diverted with this journey. I found in the low grounds hares, as I thought them to be, and foxes, but they differed greatly from all the other kinds I had met with, nor could I satisfy myself to eat them, though I killed several. But I had no need to be venturous, for I had no want of food, and that which was very good too, especially these three sorts, viz. goats, pigeons, and turtle, or tortoise, which, added to my grapes, Leadenhall Market could not have furnished a table better than I, in proportion to the company. And though my case was deplorable enough, yet I had great cause for thankfulness, and that I was not driven to any extremities for food, but rather plenty, even to dainties. I never travelled in this journey above two miles outright in a day, or thereabouts.
car swim marine ear nurse crane economic sun

N.6

with a row of stakes, set upright in the ground, either from one tree to another, or so as no wild creature could come at me without waking me. As soon as I came to the seashore, I was surprised to see that I had taken up my lot on the worst side of the island, for here indeed the shore was covered with innumerable turtles; whereas, on the other side, I found but three in a year and a half. Here was also an infinite number of fowls of many kinds, some of which I had seen, and some which I had not seen before, and many of them very good meat, but such as I knew not the names of, except those called penguins. I could have shot as many as I pleased, but was very sparing of my ruin cove examine rain swan ease conserve move

N.8

of the island, yet it was with much more difficulty that I could come near them, the country being flat and even, and they saw me much sooner than when I was on the hill. I confess this side of the country was much pleasanter than mine; but yet I had not the least inclination to remove, for as I was fixed in my habitation, it became natural to me, and I seemed all the while I was here to be as it were upon a journey, and from home. However, I travelled along the shore of the sea towards the east, I suppose about twelve miles, and then setting up a great pole nave rim common assess rinse swarm cocoon car

b

Figure 6.1 The standard methods of assessing (*a*) distance and (*b*) near vision. On the Snellen chart (*a*) note that the letters not only decrease from the top in height but also in the thickness of the strokes.

a

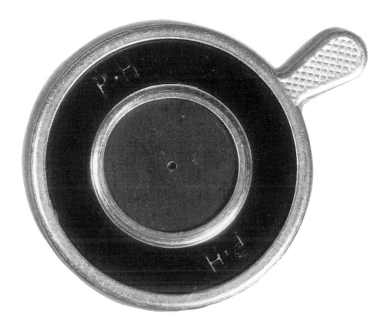

Figure 6.2 The pinhole test. The distance vision is assessed with the disc held close or in front of the distance spectacle correction.

American and European respectively. Cruder methods of assessing what vision remains in the eye consist of first asking the patient to count fingers at a distance of 1 metre, failing this to detect the movement of a hand and, finally, to perceive light shone on the eye. It is only when the patient has no perception of light that we can say that an eye is truly ophthalmologically blind.

Assessing near vision

The eyes should be tested for near vision with the patient wearing reading spectacles, if applicable. A special near vision chart is used. The conventional standard types are designated in one of two ways, J.1 and J.2, etc, or N.5, N.6, etc (Figure 6.1b). The denomination of the smallest type a patient can read at comfortable reading distance is recorded for each eye tested separately. J.1(N.5) is the standard of normal near vision.

Routine examination of the eyes by the non-specialist

An initial general inspection is carried out of the eyelids, their position, any inflammatory signs or any localized swellings. The white of the eye is checked for the presence of engorged conjunctival blood vessels. The eyeball itself is examined in two stages:

1 The anterior segment, that is, the front of the eye

2 The posterior compartment, the fundus or depths, that is, the back of the eye.

Examining the front of the eye

As far as the anterior segment is concerned, the most important point to remember is that the examining light must be focused on the part of the eye to be inspected, for example, the cornea.

Most ophthalmoscopes are unhelpful for this examination and a simple inspection torch with a focusing bulb may be much more valuable. The examination is even more informative if some form of magnification is used, such as a cheap jeweller's loupe (Figure 6.3).

The non-specialist examining the anterior segment for some possible cause of the visual defect should pay particular attention to the clarity of the cornea, to any obvious abnormality of the pupillary region of the lens and to the pupil size and reactions.

The last often results in a major distinction between those conditions which affect the clarity of the retinal image and those due to other causes of defective vision. In the former, the

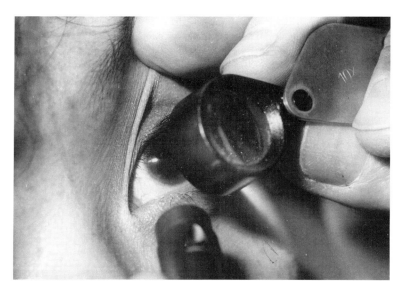

Figure 6.3 Examination of the anterior segment of the eye with simple magnification, a jeweller's loupe. It is essential when inspecting the front of the eye to use a focused source of illumination. The simple ophthalmoscope light is usually not adequate.

pupil's reaction to light is unaffected. If the pupils, both of the examined and of the fellow eye, fail to react to light shone on them, this suggests that the cause of the visual defect is to be found in some abnormality of the retina or visual pathway.

Any abnormality of the anterior segment of the eye found by these simple examination techniques indicates that the patient should be referred for slit-lamp examination by an ophthalmologist.

Examining the back of the eye—the technique of ophthalmoscopy

The fundus of the eye is the view obtained by the ophthalmoscope (Figure 6.4), a complex and difficult instrument to learn how to use. Ophthalmoscopy depends on the principle discovered by Helmholtz, that is, that inspection of the retina is possible as long as the observation is directed along the line of the entering and therefore emerging rays of light.

The only way to become an accomplished user of the ophthalmoscope is to practise repeatedly with a good instrument. Once the skill is acquired, it has great value in determining the source of defective vision. It brings into its purview such important causes as opacification of the media, retinal disease and pathology of the optic nerve, as well as providing a light with which to test pupil reaction.

The image inspected is at optical infinity, not at the apparently short 50 mm (2 inches) away. The latter mistaken notion often causes the novice to try to converge the eyes to a close distance. In doing so, the sight hole of the ophthalmoscope may be missed and the novice inappropriately accommodates for near vision, thus blurring the view.

The trick is to learn to relax both convergence and accommodation and to ignore the image from the eye not being used for the examination. Experienced ophthalmoscopists can simply ignore this mentally, but the beginner may find it advantageous purposely to close his unused eye or to cover it with his hand.

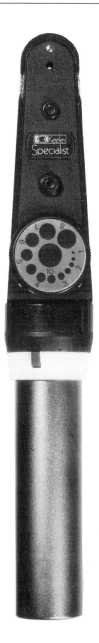

Figure 6.4 The ophthalmoscope.

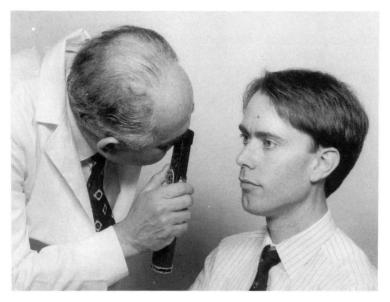

Figure 6.5   Ophthalmoscopy.

The ophthalmoscope incorporates a series of lenses that can be interposed in the view so as to take into account the optical state of the subject and of the examiner. If both eyes are optically normal, no lens is required — '0' on the ophthalmoscope dial.

Even unfocused, the observer will see a red glow through the pupil of the normal eye. This red reflex originates from blood in the choroid coming back through transparent retina and ocular media. Any substantial reduction of the red reflex, or interference with part of it, suggests opacification of the media and makes the examination difficult. If the media are normal, the appropriate adjustment of the lens dial will show a clear view of the retinal detail and of the optic nerve head.

The examiner should first ask the patient to gaze steadily horizontally ahead at a distant object, and then the eye is examined about 15 degrees outwards from the line of gaze (Figure 6.5). In this way the optic disc, which is somewhat medial to the true geometrical posterior pole of the eye, can be properly viewed. If the disc is not immediately seen, a retinal vessel will soon be picked up. This can then be followed to the optic disc, which is always examined first.

The examiner uses his right eye for the patient's right eye, and his left for the patient's left. The instrument should be held close to and in a fixed relationship to the examiner's eye so that the examiner and instrument move as one.

When using the ophthalmoscope, four elements are examined, the first three being of particular importance in cases of disturbed vision:

- The optic disc

- The emerging retinal blood vessels

- The macula

- The periphery of the retina.

The optic disc   A normal optic disc as seen through the ophthalmoscope is shown in Figure 6.6. The features of the optic disc to be noted are:

1 The clarity of the disc's edges and whether they are well defined, blurred or swollen (papilloedema), as illustrated in Figure 6.7

2 The colour of the disc, that is, whether it is pale (optic atrophy) either totally or in one part, for example, only the outer part, indicating 'temporal pallor' (Figure 6.8)

3 The presence or absence of a cup and, if present, its size and whether it approaches the true edge of the optic disc (Figures 6.9 and 6.10).

The emerging retinal blood vessels   The retinal blood vessels should be examined for their pattern and patency and, if a cup is present, for their change in direction as they enter the cup. The vessels are then followed out into the periphery in all four directions—upper and lower temporal, lower and upper nasal. The features that should be particularly noted are the arterial calibre and reflexes from the walls, the arteriovenous crossings and any pathology within or alongside the vessels (emboli, haemorrhages, or exudates).

The macula   As noted, the 'business end' of the retina is the macula. To inspect this the examiner

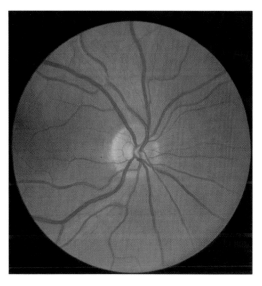

Figure 6.6   The normal optic disc. The edges are clearly defined and the temporal edge often has a slight pigmentation near by. The pattern of the vessels is characteristic. The arterioles are lighter in colour and narrower in calibre than the venous tributaries. All the vessels cross the margins of the disc without any significant alteration in direction.

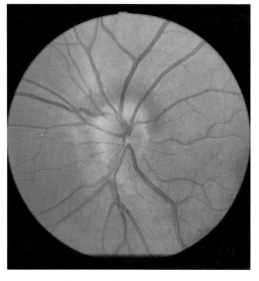

Figure 6.7   Blurred edges to the optic disc – early papilloedema.

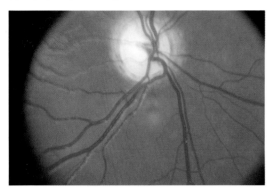

Figure 6.8   Optic atrophy. The disc is very much paler than its normal pink colour and the atrophy shown here is ischaemic, as shown by the marked sheathing of one of the branches of the inferior temporal retinal arteriole.

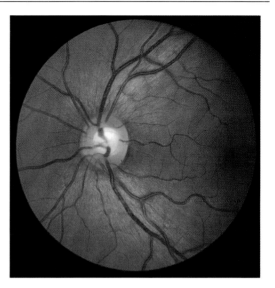

Figure 6.9   A normal disc showing a well defined, moderate-sized physiological cup. The dusky hue of the retina is characteristic of patients with heavily pigmented skin.

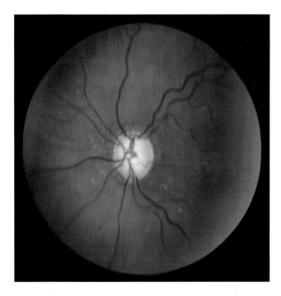

Figure 6.10   A glaucomatous disc. The cup extends virtually to the edge of the disc proper where the vessel drops backwards sharply and may appear discontinuous.

must either look at the area outward (temporally) from the disc, or ask the patient to look at the light of the ophthalmoscope. Unfortunately this introduces two technical problems. First, the cornea throws light back into the ophthalmoscope, dazzling the examiner and, second, the pupil becomes smaller.

It is no wonder that even the ophthalmologist cannot always give an opinion about the macula without the pupil being dilated by drugs. The novice should therefore not feel frustrated by being unable to see any macular pathology (unless very gross), when the pupil is not dilated. One point to remember is that if the eye has suffered any severe loss of vision, it is possible that the pupil will not contract well, or at all, and this can make the examination easier.

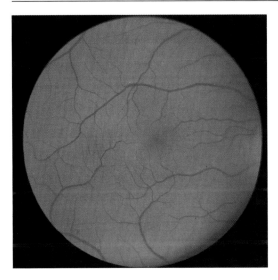

Figure 6.11 The normal macula of a right eye. The edge of the disc can be seen at the right of the picture. Note that the macular area itself is substantially free of vessels but that numerous branches of the main vessels are directed towards it.

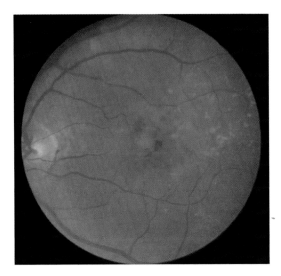

Figure 6.12 Senile macular degeneration. Irregular white and pigmented small blotches are visible in what is normally a featureless area of the fundus.

The macula is normally featureless, save for a bright pinpoint light reflex from the fovea (Figure 6.11). Abnormality may be indicated by haemorrhages or white patches or pigment clumps (Figure 6.12).

Owing to the technical difficulty in viewing the macula with an undilated pupil, any systematic examination should include the instillation of mydriatic (pupil-dilating) drops, typically cyclopentolate (1 per cent). This facilitates the inspection of the macula, but also of the retinal periphery. After completing the examination, the mydriasis should be reversed by pilocarpine (1 per cent) drops.

In very rare instances, dilatation of the pupil by drops may precipitate closed angle glaucoma (see Chapter 13), but this is very unlikely to occur if, before using such drops, the examiner is satisfied that the anterior chamber is not unduly shallow.

The periphery of the retina By asking the patient to look in different directions, the periphery of the retina may be inspected. The important changes found here relate particularly to retinal holes and detachments, and to some fine vessel changes.

Using the ophthalmoscope to detect media opacities As noted, opacification of the media interferes with the ophthalmoscope view. In such cases, the ophthalmoscope may help to diagnose precisely which structure is affected. Obviously, if any one of the media is totally opaque, then no reflex is obtained. If the red reflex is only partially obscured, the ophthalmoscope can be focused to a level in front of the retina—even to the level of the pupil—by interposing convex lenses, using the lens dial. Immature (incomplete) cataract may be outlined clearly as a black opacity which the red reflex fails to transilluminate as it returns from the fundus (Figure 6.13). Such lens opacities form stationary patterns. Opacities in the vitreous are usually not fixed and therefore, with the ophthalmoscope appropriately focused, they are seen as mobile black objects.

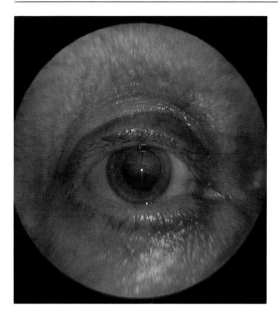

Figure 6.13 The appearance of opacities of the media, as seen by the ophthalmoscope when it is focused anterior to the retina, in this case at the level of the pupil and lens. A case of moderate cortical cataract.

Finally, it should be appreciated by those not trained in certain technical aspects of eye examination that it is sometimes impossible to reach a firm diagnosis in cases of defective vision. For this reason the problem of referral is an important one, and may of course arise even when a definitive diagnosis has been made.

REFERRAL

Referral for a further opinion on patients with visual difficulty may originate from a number of different sources such as family practitioners, opticians and optometrists, and other medical specialists.

It should be remembered that self-referral to an optician or optometrist is the common first step for a patient with a visual problem in many countries of the world. Since it is likely that the condition is an optical one and can be diagnosed and treated by the optician, this first step by the patient is usually quite satisfactory, circumventing any medical involvement. If any non-optical condition is discovered, either as the cause of the patient's complaint or coincidentally, it is the optician's professional duty to refer the patient back to his or her general practitioner, or in an emergency to an ophthalmologist.

If a patient initially seeks the advice of a medical practitioner who is not an ophthalmologist on some visual problem, and referral to an eye specialist is deemed to be advisable, two questions must be answered:

1 Should the referral be for a medical or a non-medical ophthalmic opinion?

2 How urgent is the referral?

Referral to an optician by the non-specialist

As far as referral to an optician is concerned, there are many circumstances where this is the logical, or perhaps only, step:

● The forty-year-old and older patient complaining of difficulty in reading

● The adolescent having difficulty seeing the blackboard, etc

● Visual disturbance due to eyestrain

● Non-acute visual complaints in any patient of whatever age, who has never worn spectacles may reasonably call for an optician's sight test.

Being trained to use the ophthalmoscope the optician or optometrist may, as noted, be more proficient than some who are medically qualified. For this reason, the optician is often the first port of call for an 'eye opinion' and provided the patient and the general practitioner realize the limitations of the opinion and management, this arrangement should work well.

Referral to an ophthalmologist

In certain cases the optician should be bypassed, and referral made directly to an ophthalmologist. For example, where there is visual disturbance in spite of a fairly recent change of spectacles, or if the patient's vision has not been satisfactorily improved by a new pair of spectacles.

It should also be borne in mind that although opticians have an important role to play in establishing or eliminating optical causes for eye complaints, such as those found in eyestrain and headaches, there are a host of eye symptoms that rarely, if ever, fall within the optician's clinical field. These would include many of the complaints enumerated in Chapters 2, 3 and 5. Indeed, in some countries of the world, for example, the USA, where there are many ophthalmologists, self-referral by the patient direct to the ophthalmologist replaces initial examination by an optician. This applies even when the complaint is an optical one.

It is also the author's opinion that at least the initial examination of all children's eyes, whether routine or for some clinical anomaly, optical or otherwise, should be by an ophthalmologist.

Urgent referral

Acute perstistent visual disturbance or loss of vision should never be referred to an optician, but forthwith for a medical opinion at perhaps the emergency department of an eye hospital, or

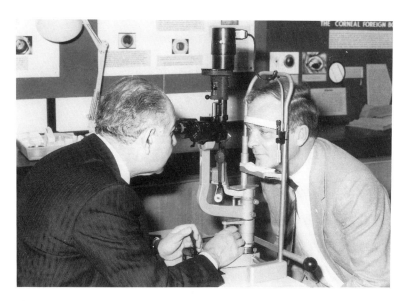

Figure 6.14 Slit-lamp examination.

of a general hosiptal where it is known there is residential ophthalmic staff.

Diagnosis by the ophthalmologist

We have already noted the paramount importance of inspection in ophthalmic diagnosis. The routine eye examinations made by the ophthalmologist are with the ophthalmoscope (see pages 35–40) and the slit-lamp.

Slit-lamp examination   The slit-lamp (Figure 6.14) is essentially an ophthalmological tool used extensively for examining the front of the eye under magnification. It is basically a low-powered binocular microscope which is used to inspect a slit-shaped beamed light accurately focused in the same plane as that of the microscope. Detailed inspection of the front of the eye including all layers of the cornea is possible under a magnification of up to forty times. In addition, the contents of the anterior chamber and the structure of the iris can be easily seen. With the pupil dilated, a substantial part of the lens and the anterior vitreous are visible.

Gonioscopy   In glaucoma sufferers, the use of a special type of contact lens—a gonioscope—

allows inspection of the anterior chamber angle and this examination is very important in distinguishing the various types of glaucoma (see pages 111–28).

Applanation tonometry is the most reliable method of measuring the ocular pressure, and this is usually carried out by slit-lamp examination.

The retina   By using a contact lens to abolish the refraction of the cornea, the slit-lamp offers the possibility of inspecting the retina. The incorporation within the contact lens of mirrors of various tilts makes possible the examination of the retinal periphery and the flat part of the ciliary body in addition to the area of the disc and the macula. This type of examination is particularly important in identifying the presence and position of retinal holes prior to procedures for treating retinal detachment.

Finally, it should be mentioned that allied to its diagnostic function, the slit-lamp used in combination with contact lenses has important therapeutic value in acting as a delivery system for laser treatment to the iris, to lens remnants after cataract extraction, or to the retina (see page 100).

Table 6.1 The non-specialist reading this book should be able to perform all that is suggested in the second column and be acquainted with the scope and limits of the examinations made by the other two groups of professionals.

Techniques	Non-specialist	Optometrist/optician	Ophthalmologist
Assessing vision	Simple assessment of visual acuity with and without spectacles for near and distance	Sight test—refraction of patient, objective and subjective tests; retinoscopy	As in Column 3
Possible optical improvement	Pinhole test	With lenses based on objective findings	As in Column 3
Examining the anterior segment of the eye	Focused torch with or without magnification	As in Column 2 plus possible slit-lamp examination	Slit-lamp examination
Examination of the fundus	Ophthalmoscopy of central retina and optic disc	Ophthalmoscopy with or without dilating the pupil	Ophthalmoscopy, usually with dilatation of the pupil
The ocular pressure	Digital tonometry (p.112)	Digital tonometry or instrumental by air tonometer or by applanation	All methods but usually by applanation
Visual field	By confrontation (p.116)	By instrumental technique (perimetry)	By perimetry
Muscle balance	Inspection of corneal reflections; cover test; ocular movements (pp.182–7)	Inspection, cover test and ocular movements with possible synoptophore examination	Similar to previous columns plus orthoptic referral
Special investigations:			
Microbiology	Yes	No	Yes
Electro-diagnostic tests	No	No	Yes
Fluorescein angiography	No	No	Yes
Ultrasound examination	No	No	Yes

PART 2: COMMON EYE CONDITIONS

The only criterion for including any particular eye condition in this section of the book is the frequency of its occurrence and the virtual certainty that the non-ophthalmologist will encounter it at some stage in his or her professional career.

Part 2 starts with an overview of optical problems, the most numerous of the causes of blurred sight. In subsequent chapters, an outline is given of the abnormalities of the eyeball. For each ocular structure the effect of the disorder on the sight is noted, any other symptoms are described, and treatment given (Chapters 7 to 13). The neighbourhood structures concerned with ocular protection are considered, and the results of failed ocular protection (injuries) reviewed (Chapters 14 to 18). Finally, the various types of incoordination of the eyes are presented (Chapter 19).

Thus it can be said that most ophthalmic conditions fall into three groups:

- Disorders of the visual apparatus; the eyeball itself and the visual pathway

- Abnormalities of the protective structures

- Disturbance of coordination of the two eyes.

This subdivision is of course to some degree artificial because the three categories are closely interrelated. The normal visual apparatus is dependent on an adequate protective mechanism, and uncoordinated eyes give rise to, but may also arise from, disorders of the visual apparatus.

In standard ophthalmology texts, the didactic approach to the description of disease usually involves a description of its aetiology, pathogenesis, diagnosis, prognosis and treatment. This has not been slavishly followed here because of the great variation in the relative clinical importance of these factors between differing eye diseases. For instance, the aetiology of cataract has little to do with its management whereas, on the contrary, the mechanism of closed angle glaucoma has a direct relevance to its treatment.

Before proceeding to short formal descriptions of the common eye conditions, it is pertinent to set down some of the main features that distinguish ophthalmic pathology and prognosis from other branches of medicine.

Pathology and ophthalmology

Whatever its relationship to diagnosis and treatment, conventional techniques of pathology are beset with difficulties in ophthalmology, as shown by the practical impossibility of biopsy, at least with respect to vital structures such as the retina.

Most pathological studies of the eyeball are necessarily the result of work on eyes removed during life, or at a post mortem. As far as the former is concerned, the indications to remove an eye, as in severe painful glaucoma, for example, make it virtually certain that gross advanced pathology is present, which tends to vitiate any conclusion about the early stages of disease. Studies from post mortem eyes are rare because the material from subjects with known ophthalmic complaints is often unavailable.

In spite of major efforts in the field of ophthalmic pathology, we remain substantially ignorant about the basic causes of many major eye diseases; for example, cataract, chronic simple glaucoma and macular disease. Limited space does not permit speculative discussion on unsolved problems, so pathology is kept to a minimum, except where it offers a direct explanation of a clinically important feature of presentation or management.

Prognosis of eye diseases

As in other branches of medicine, prognosis will depend on the natural course of the disease process and its response to treatment. It is, however, important to remember that when looking for improvement in the sight, the prognosis is inevitably overshadowed by the nature of the particular affected structure of the eye concerned. There is always a possibility of improvement in vision if the defect is one concerning the quality of the retinal image, but sight or visual field lost due to a destructive disease in the retina or in the visual pathway is likely to be permanent. Because of the embryological central nervous origin of these tissues, regeneration is impossible.

Even in those tissues of the visual apparatus subserving the retinal image, recovery from active disease may not be accompanied by a full return of function. An example of this is scarring of the cornea once a corneal ulcer has healed, or irreversible opacity of the lens from trauma. The disorganization, to a greater or lesser degree, of one of the ocular media during the period of the active process can be succeeded by such an irregular optical condition that management by standard optical methods is impossible. However, as noted, in the vast majority of cases where the retinal image is indistinct, the ocular media are perfectly healthy. (Chapter 7 describes these optical defects.)

7 Optical problems and correction of optical errors

Optical abnormalities of the eyes, the refractive errors, are the principal cause of blurred vision. Before considering the refractive errors, the normal optical state of the eye is discussed.

The normal optical state of the eye

Normal distance vision

An optically normal **emmetropic** eye focuses parallel rays of light as a point image on the retina. Consequently a distance point object forms a point image that will be seen clearly when the eye is directed so that the image falls on the macula.

Most of the focusing takes place at the surface of the cornea, due to its curvature and because of the large change of refractive index between air and corneal substance. The lens of the eye further modifies the path of the rays, which are already converging owing to the refraction by the cornea, so that they converge even more and focus on the retina (Figure 7.1).

Normal near vision

When a close object is viewed, the rays reaching the eye are diverging. Such near vision stimulates the process of accommodation. The shape

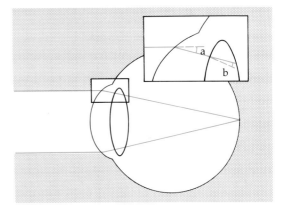

Figure 7.1 The focusing mechanism of an optically normal – emmetropic – eye. Note that most of the refraction takes place at the cornea, the lens of the eye playing a minor but very important part (i.e., angle *a* is greater than angle *b*).

of the lens of the eye becomes more convex and the lens can then converge the rays to focus on the retina. This process is brought about by the contraction of the ciliary muscle, induced by parasympathetic nerves which run with the IIIrd cranial nerve, the oculomotor. The lens is suspended under tension from the ciliary body,

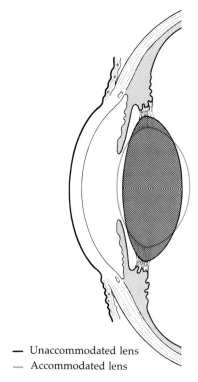

— Unaccommodated lens
— Accommodated lens

Figure 7.2 The mechanism of accommodation.

within which is found the ciliary muscle. When the muscle contracts, the tension decreases to allow the lens to bulge along its axis (Figure 7.2).

The measurement of the optical state — refracting the patient

As we have noted in Part 1, this procedure, also known as a sight test, conducted by a specialist, consists of three components:

1 An assessment of the patient's vision, without any optical aid

2 Measurement of the optical state of the eyes—objective refraction

3 Reassessment of the visual acuity of the eyes with the aid of any lenses indicated by the above measurement—subjective refraction.

Assessment of the patient's unaided vision This involves testing each eye separately, without any optical aid and without any optical correction that the patient is currently using (see page 31). The standard of vision is the uncorrected visual acuity.

Measurement of the optical state of the eyes— objective refraction This procedure, known as retinoscopy, is usually carried out by specialists, opticians or ophthalmologists (note that retinoscopy is different from ophthalmoscopy—see Chapter 6).

In retinoscopy, the direction of the movement of a light across the eye is compared to the direction of the movement of the light reflex emerging from the pupil. The emerging light moves in the same or opposite direction to the external movement, according to the optical condition of the eye. Lenses of varying strengths are interposed until one is found with which the movement in the pupil is abolished, so that it becomes impossible to tell whether the emerging light is moving with or against the external light. From the power of the lens producing this neutralization point, an estimate can be made of the optical state of the eye.

The objective examination of the optical state can now be performed by automated computerized instruments, but this has not yet gained universal acceptance, partly owing to its expense.

Reassessment of the visual acuity The final element of a sight test is the reassessment of the visual acuity of the eyes using the optical aids indicated by the objective refraction. This element is known as subjective refraction and gives the corrected visual acuity.

The refractive errors

The optical coordination of the normal eye depends on the curvatures and separation of the refracting surfaces, as well as the refractive indices of the clear media between the surfaces. In the usual refractive errors, the commonest anomaly is an incorrect distance of the plane of focus — the retina.

The following refractive errors are considered:

- Myopia
- Hypermetropia
- Presbyopia
- Astigmatism
- Anisometropia.

Myopia

In myopia (the terms short sightedness or near sight are most commonly used by the layman)

the retina is behind the plane of focus, that is, the eye is optically too long. Note that the myopic eye is 'long' but produces short sightedness — the inability to see distant objects clearly (Figure 7.3). The condition may, and sometimes does, arise because the optical power of the cornea and lens are greater than usual. In most cases the eye is actually physically longer than average. The statistically average length of an optically normal eye is about 24 mm (just less than 1 in). In high myopia, the eye may be as much as 7 or 8 mm longer than this.

Symptoms   The myope has a 'far point' beyond which no object can be seen clearly; objects nearer than the far point can be focused by accommodation.

Myopia is rarely congenital. Much more commonly, it commences at about the age of ten years, or slightly older. The usual initial complaint is difficulty in seeing the blackboard at school, or of having to sit close to the television. Once a 'school myope' is discovered, and spectacles prescribed, it is quite usual for the strength of the myopic correction to need to be increased progressively over the teenage years. In the vast majority of cases the correction required for distance vision is attained by the age of twenty-one years in males and slightly younger in females, and will remain unaltered more or less indefinitely.

The precise cause of myopia   is unknown, but there are definite familial and racial predispositions. The most important unresolved question is the relation of 'excessive' reading to the genesis and progression of the condition. It has been suggested that the 'intellectual habit' is in the genes and that the 'reading' produces the myopia, thus negating the idea that myopia itself is inherited, at least in some cases.

Optical correction of myopia   is by concave lenses of such a power that the parallel rays are made to diverge so they apparently arise from the far point (Figure 7.4). The lens power is

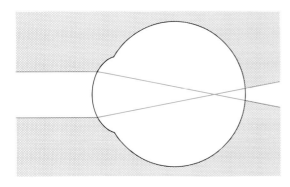

Figure 7.3   Myopia. Parallel rays of light focus in front of the retina.

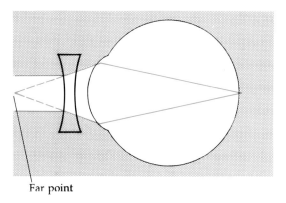

Far point

Figure 7.4   The correction of myopia. A concave lens is used to make the parallel rays appear to diverge from the far point.

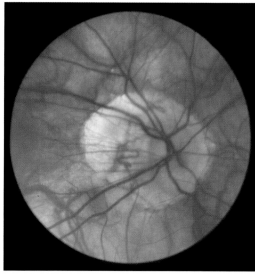

a

measured in dioptres (a dioptre being the reciprocal of the focal length in metres).

Myopia of any significant degree, perhaps greater than 2 dioptre, is *par excellence* the condition requiring the constant wearing of an optical correction (usually spectacles) for clear distance vision. It is also the main indication for the wearing of contact lenses as a cosmetically more acceptable alternative. There are of course other reasons for preferring contact lenses, and these are discussed on pages 57–60.

Associations of myopia   Higher degrees of myopia (over about 8 dioptre) are associated with two important conditions: macular degeneration and retinal detachment.

1 **Macular degeneration**   This is often considered to be a stretching phenomenon associated with the enlargement and elongation of the eyeball, especially in its posterior segment (Figure 7.5). The condition may

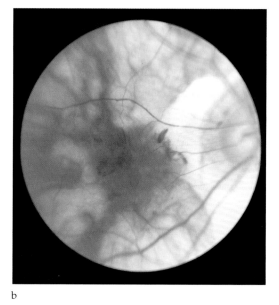

b

Figure 7.5   Stretching changes at the posterior pole of highly myopic eyes: (*a*) shows a large temporal crescent extending towards the macula; (*b*) shows a haemorrhagic area at the macula itself, with pigmentation. The white area between the disc and the macula is additional evidence of myopic stretching associated with the increased size of the eyeball.

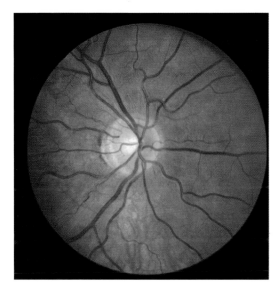

Figure 7.6 A small myopic crescent such as might occur in a myope of fairly low degree, characteristically on the temporal side of the disc.

cause a defect of vision that is not correctable with spectacles. Even in lower degrees of myopia a characteristic change may be seen with the ophthalmoscope (the myopic crescent temporal to the optic disc, as shown in Figure 7.6), but this is not associated with visual loss.

2 **Retinal detachment** The stretching changes that affect the retina in the posterior part of the eyeball may be matched by similar pathology in the retinal periphery. There may also be an actual mechanical tear, or tears, through which fluid may pass from the rather degenerate vitreous to separate the retina from the choroid, thus producing a retinal detachment. In fact, some degree of degeneration of the vitreous is a feature of most myopic eyes, whatever the degree of the optical error, and the complaint of spots

in the vision is a frequent one (see Chapter 11 for more details).

The fundus changes in high myopia are sometimes difficult to see for the examiner inexperienced in the use of the ophthalmoscope. A useful tip is to remember that, for a high myope, it is best to examine the fundus through the patient's own spectacles rather than to try focusing on the fundus by altering the lenses of the ophthalmoscope itself.

Surgery for myopia Of recent years, operations have been devised to counteract myopia by decreasing the curvature of the cornea. Multiple partial thickness radial incisions are made — radial keratotomy. The scarring that occurs produces a less convex surface. Although a now widely accepted procedure, it is still in a somewhat tentative phase, the results being not entirely predictable. The use of the laser for the same purpose is still largely experimental at present.

Other associations of myopia Myopia occurring in middle life or old age may be a sign of an organic change in the lens of the eye. The prime suspects are diabetes or senile cataract. One condition which virtually never occurs in a lifelong myope is acute (closed angle) glaucoma, the angle of the anterior chamber in the myopia usually being so wide as to preclude its ever closing.

Hypermetropia

In this condition the focus falls behind the retina (Figure 7.7). In fact, here, the eye is too short, and in higher degrees of hypermetropia the eye is often physically small.

The alternative terms for hypermetropia are 'far sight' or 'long sight', but unfortunately these are often used by patients and family practitioners to describe optical normality. The confusion arises from the fact that if hypermetropes have

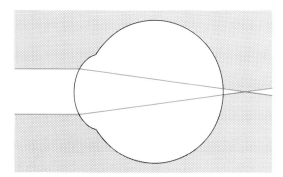

Figure 7.7 Hypermetropia. Parallel rays of light focus behind the retina.

any symptoms at all, they are predominantly difficulties with reading and close work, and there is little interference with distance vision.

Symptoms Whether a hypermetrope has any symptoms depends on the eye's power of accommodation (Figure 7.8). Of course the optically normal eye does not use any accommodation for distance. But if the hypermetrope accommodates

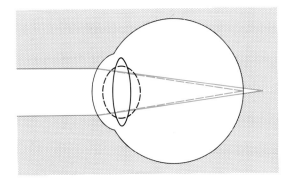

Figure 7.8 The correction of hypermetropia by accommodation, which is used here even for distance vision.

for distance vision, making the lens more powerfully converging, distant objects can be clearly focused on the retina.

Accommodation is an involuntary function, so the subject is unaware he is exerting accommodation, and therefore no symptoms occur. Furthermore, if the hypermetrope has an abundance of accommodation, the extra accommodative power required for close vision may be available and, even in that function, symptoms will not arise. However, if the degree of hypermetropia is high and the available accommodation inadequate, blurring of close vision may occur.

The most pertinent fact about accommodation is that its power is age-related. Even in an optically normal person (the emmetrope) there is a steady decline of accommodative power with age. In the forty to forty-five age group the 'near point', which is the closest point at which an object can be clearly seen, has receded to an uncomfortable arm's length. To the hypermetrope this decline in accommodation brings reading difficulties at an earlier period, even at a much earlier age, if the degree of optical error is large.

During childhood, many hypermetropes are undetected and untroubled for near and distance vision. It also appears that a vast majority of us are born with hypermetropia to some degree, and this then declines progressively through childhood. In some, this situation actually proceeds to a myopic error in the teenage years.

As mentioned, if a hypermetrope has any symptoms at all they will initially be for close work. It should be remembered, however, that accommodation eventually declines to nothing in the late fifties age group, when the hypermetrope not only fails to accommodate for close work but cannot clearly focus even distant objects. Many elderly hypermetropes, who had no need for spectacles at all in early life, often need correction for both distance and near vision.

Apart from actual blurring of vision for close work, the unconsciously provoked excessive accommodation may lead to symptoms of eyestrain, headaches, pain in the eyes and congested eyes (see Chapter 4).

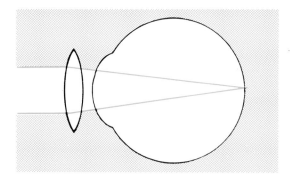

Figure 7.9 The correction of hypermetropia by a convex lens.

Optical correction of hypermetropia The type of lens needed to correct hypermetropia is convex and the power required is usually sufficient to replace the inadequacy of the patient's own accommodation (Figure 7.9). The patient's spectacles may be required only for close work, and this is probably the reason why the wearing of contact lenses is far less widespread for this condition than for myopia.

Associations of hypermetropia There is often nothing particularly characteristic about the retinal appearance in hypermetropia. In fact, the optic disc often looks, and actually may be, slightly smaller than in an optically normal subject. The crowding of the retinal nerve fibres collecting here to form the optic nerve may give a blurred appearance to the disc edge. This is sometimes misdiagnosed as papilloedema (see Chapter 23) and is termed 'pseudo papillo edema'; the veins in the hypermetrope may be tortuous but are not dilated and, if anything, appear quite the opposite. True papilloedema is associated with venous congestion.

In a small number of cases, important organic conditions may be encountered with hypermetropia. In particular two conditions are worthy of note:

1 **Concomitant convergent strabismus** (squint) in children. This arises from a disturbed relationship between the convergence of the two eyes needed to view a near object, and the excessive accommodation needed by the hypermetropic eyes in order to see it clearly (see also Chapter 19).

2 **Closed angle glaucoma** The condition springs from the smallness of the eye in many hypermetropic patients. The smallness is further illustrated by the shallow anterior chamber and the chamber angle being narrow. The iris is closer to the cornea and, in conditions where the pupil dilates, it bunches up and may block the anterior chamber angle, blocking the outflow of aqueous humour.

As noted, hypermetropia is a condition usually present from early life, though the age at which symptoms arise (and therefore at which the condition is discovered) is variable. The development of hypermetropia in a patient previously known to be optically normal occurs most frequently following cataract surgery during which an intraocular lens is not implanted. This is the optical condition known as aphakia. More rarely, an optical shortening of the eye may be a sign of swelling of the macula or indentation of the globe caused by orbital pressure.

Presbyopia

This term is used to describe the condition in which patients experience difficulty with close work owing to the decline of accommodation with age. Close print such as in a newspaper or telephone directory has to be held farther away. This condition typically commences in patients over forty years of age. Everybody becomes presbyopic, whether previously emmetropic, myopic or hypermetropic.

1 The emmetrope who has never previously needed any optical aid for distance or near vision may be shocked to discover that his unaided vision is becoming blurred for reading.

2 The myope, in attempting to read with distance correcting spectacles, experiences the same symptoms as the emmetrope.

3 The hypermetrope experiences these difficulties earlier in life (see page 52).

Optical correction of presbyopia The correction for difficulty in reading is usually a convex (converging) lens or a weaker concave one used for close work (Figure 7.10). The following points are worthy of note:

1 The **emmetrope** will find that his reading correction actually blurs his distance sight. Hence the need to wear spectacles for close work only, or alternatively half spectacles, which allow clear unaided distance vision over the top of the correction.

2 The correction for the **myope** is achieved either by using a weaker concave lens, or indeed using no lens at all. Thus, some myopes of presbyopic age simply take off their distance spectacles in order to read.

3 For **hypermetropes** developing presbyopia, a stronger convex lens is needed for near than for distance vision.

4 For the **presbyope** who needs some kind of distance correction, either constantly or intermittently, the near correction can be incorporated in the lower segment of the spectacle glass as a bifocal lens. This saves the individual having to change from one pair of spectacles to another. Unfortunately, however, some people are unable to tolerate bifocals because they find that they experience difficulty in going down steps or

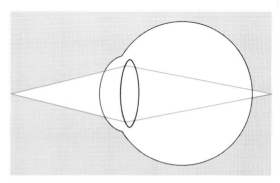

a

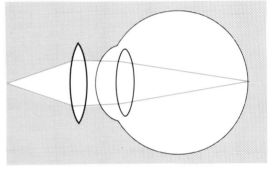

b

Figure 7.10 (*a*) Presbyopia. If the lens cannot accommodate adequately, a near object will not be focused clearly on the retina. (*b*) In these circumstances a convex lens is needed for reading and close work.

stepping off kerbs. In looking down, they are using the close vision section of the lens rather than the distance vision section. Additionally, the sharp change of focus between the two corrections in bifocals can sometimes cause dizziness.

The newer varifocal spectacles that are now available are graded steadily from distance to near vision and give a variable intermediate focus, which is much appreciated by many patients.

The power of the near correction required in presbyopia increases between the ages of forty-five and fifty-five years. Every two or three years the initial symptoms—blurred vision on reading, especially in bad light, or having to push the print farther away—will recur even when the individual is using the current spectacle prescription. Finally, in the late fifties, the reading correction stabilizes and any further optical change is minimal.

Astigmatism

Astigmatism is a common optical anomaly which can coexist with myopia or hypermetropia. Optically, the condition is what its name implies, no point image being formed by the eye when a point object is viewed.

Astigmatism arises from the dissimilarity of the optical condition of the eye in differing planes, particularly in the refraction by the cornea (Figure 7.11). Essentially, the curvature of the cornea is ovular, more marked in one plane (meridian) than the other.

Symptoms   A mild degree of astigmatism may not give rise to any symptoms. If more marked, the condition results in blurred vision that may be tolerable or go unnoticed for distance vision, but gives rise to reading difficulties. The reason for this is that some parts of a letter may be more clearly focused than others, giving rise to problems of identification. Apart from illegibility, the frustrating attempt to focus the astigmatic eye may cause eyestrain.

Optical correction of astigmatism is achieved by incorporating a cylindrical lens into the spectacle glass, which also corrects the 'spherical' error of hypermetropia or myopia. The orientation of the cylindrical correction must match up to the orientation of the astigmatic error of the eye. A typical compound astigmatic correction is illustrated in Figure 7.12.

Anisometropia

The term anisometropia is used to describe the optical condition where a patient's two eyes

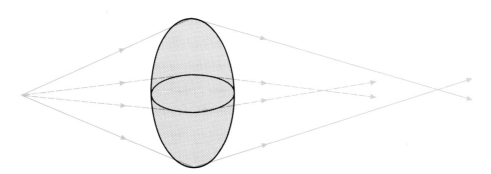

Figure 7.11   The optics of astigmatism. The continuous line is the optical condition in the vertical plane; the broken line that in the horizontal plane.

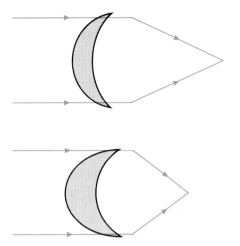

Figure 7.12   The focusing in different planes by an astigmatic lens, which is of different convexity in its two principal meridia: *above*, the horizontal meridian; *below*, the vertical meridian. Such a lens may be employed to correct the optical error produced by a cornea that is flatter in the vertical meridian than it is in the horizontal.

have markedly differing refractive errors, one eye perhaps even being optically normal, or emmetropic.

A peculiar problem arises if the eyes have this disparity from birth or early life; with lenses it may be impossible fully to correct the vision of the eye with the higher refractive error. This is because the brain has become used to suppressing the blurred, or more blurred, image so that the sight is defective even when a clearly focused retinal image is provided. This is a form of lazy eye (amblyopia) which is similar to that occurring in squint (see Chapter 19). In squint, the purpose of the suppression is simply to prevent intrusion into consciousness of the two dissimilar images. In anisometropia, the suppression avoids the nuisance of blurred vision from one of the eyes.

If this situation is recognized in early life, the corrected vision of the amblyopic eye will often improve in response to occlusion of the good eye. Anisometropia is therefore an important condition to recognize during the routine checking of a pre-school child's vision, as well as during the school years. In fact an anisometrope may have no symptoms and may be unaware that the image of one eye is blurred.

Correction of refractive errors

Spectacles

The supply of spectacles is usually carried out by opticians or optometrists, either ophthalmic or dispensing (see Chapter 6).

The manufacture of spectacles, as with contact lenses, is an integral part of the optical industry. Spectacle lenses are made either of glass or of plastic, the latter being lighter to wear but more liable to be scratched. The actual shaping of spectacle lenses to a frame of the patient's choice is normally carried out by the manufacturer, who works to the optical requirements of the patient's prescription and to certain measurements of the patient's face, as taken by the optician. These measurements ensure that the spectacles are comfortable and stable on the bridge of the patient's nose, along the temple and behind the ears, and that the lenses are properly mounted, their centres opposite the centres of the respective pupils, with their posterior surfaces at an appropriate distance from the eye.

In some countries, spectacles are available without prescription simply as a commercial article and without the involvement of an optician or optometrist. This situation has generally arisen in response to the need for reading spectacles, presbyopia, an almost universal visual problem experienced in middle age. While counter dispensing is often deprecated, little harm can result as long as the limitations of this practice are fully realized. What the patient who chooses spectacles is doing is giving him or herself a kind of subjective sight test (see Chapter 6), which is of course only part of a complete eye examination. Obviously some ophthalmic pathology may be ignored or missed, but even if the spectacles are incorrect by professional standards, they are likely to be simply convex spherical lenses used for presbyopia. These will do no harm if, as is likely, the eyes are in all other respects quite healthy. The myth of 'wrong spectacles ruining the eyes' is quite fallacious in an adult. If the wrong spectacles are used, the wearer will not see properly, or will develop eyestrain or headaches, but no permanent ill-effect will be experienced. All the patient has to do is stop using the offending spectacles and go for a professional sight test.

In children, however, the situation is not the same. The improvement in vision of an amblyopic or lazy eye (see Chapter 19) may be delayed and even permanently prevented by the wearing of incorrect spectacles.

Tinted glasses There are many ophthalmic conditions in which reduction in the amount of light reaching the eye is desirable. Acute inflammation of the anterior segment, for example, iritis, or treatment of conditions with pupil-dilating drugs, may be associated with photophobia.

The visual interference caused by partial cataract may be aggravated by the small pupil occurring in bright illumination. All these cases may be helped by the wearing of dark glasses.

In addition, some cases of defective ocular pigmentation, of extreme degree in albinism but occurring to some extent in the fair complexioned, may also warrant reduction in light volume.

In many cases, however, claimed dislike of the light is psychogenic; if not, the wearing of tinted glasses is simply a cosmetic aid. This is not to say that some specific activities such as prolonged exposure to bright sunlight do not also require some form of tinted glass, perhaps incorporating the patient's optical correction. In addition, some forms of tinted glass are designed specifically to exclude particular radiations such as infra red or ultra violet (in sunbeds and so on).

Tinted glasses are manufactured either using materials that are themselves tinted or by coating the correction lenses.

Problems with spectacles Although uncommon, many things can go wrong with the provision of spectacles. For example, the sight testing may be inaccurate or the wrong prescription may be made up, or the frame may be ill-fitting. Furthermore, it is important to ensure that the patient, optician and family practitioner are aware of the limitations of the sight test.

If, with newly dispensed spectacles, the patient's sight is poor in one or the other eye, the patient should return to whoever carried out the sight test. That examiner must then be satisfied as to the cause of the poor sight and, where appropriate, seek further advice.

Contact lenses

The use of a lens closely applied to the eye, a contact lens, has several obvious advantages:

1 Cosmetically, contact lenses may be more acceptable to the patient than spectacles.

2 The contact lens usually moves with the eyeball so that the quality of optical correction it gives is fairly uniform, whatever the direction of the gaze. This is particularly of value with all high refractive errors because the optical quality of powerful spectacle lenses is very poor outside a small central area, when the object looked at becomes distorted in shape and direction.

3 High myopes or aphakic patients (patients who have had cataract surgery) find contact lenses particularly beneficial. With them they get a more normal retinal image size than with the thick spectacles they would otherwise have to use. The image is larger than that achieved with spectacles in a myope and smaller in the high hypermetrope (for example, the aphakic).

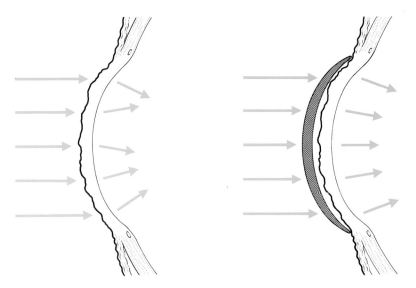

Figure 7.13   How a contact lens may be helpful in improving vision when the corneal surface is irregular.

4 If the corneal surface is irregular, contact lenses can be specifically advantageous because the optical front surface of the eye becomes effectively that of the front surface of the contact lens (Figure 7.13).

Types of contact lenses

The main differences between the various types of contact lenses are the materials they are made of, and the extent to which they cover the eye. Contact lenses generally fall into two groups: hard and soft.

Hard lenses are rigid lenses made of Perspex, or from one of a number of gas-permeable plastics. Perspex is the classical material used for hard lenses, though it can give rise to an interference with the corneal metabolism by occluding the surface. This can lead to stagnation in the tear film between the lens and the cornea, depleting particularly the oxygen supply. This was a more frequent problem with the older, and now much less common, type of haptic or scleral lens which covered not only the cornea, but also a large part of the white of the eye. It is much less of a problem with a small corneal lens, which is often well tolerated by the wearer (Figure 7.14). Lenses made of gas-permeable plastic are believed to be better tolerated. Hard lenses need to be removed, cleaned and replaced daily.

Soft lenses   The rapid growth in the production of soft contact lenses made, in many instances, of hydrophilic chemical derivatives of the hard lens material, bids to replace the hard lens for many purposes. There are, however, still difficulties with their durability and sterilization. Boiling or soaking in special chemical solutions are commonly used.

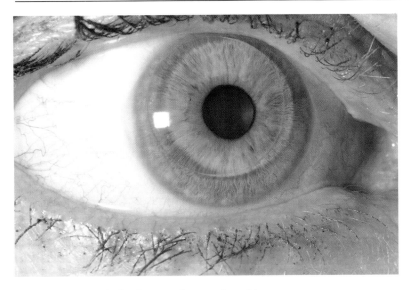

Figure 7.14   A rigid – hard – corneal contact lens. Note
that its diameter is less than that of the cornea.

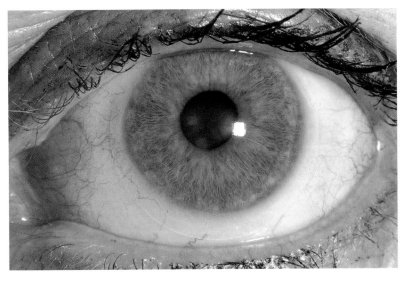

Figure 7.15   A non-rigid – soft – contact lens. Note
that the edge of the lens extends over on to the white
of the eye.

The soft lens usually slightly overlaps the corneoscleral junction (Figure 7.15), but although they are larger than the hard, corneal lens, they are often more comfortable. At present, owing to their soft physical characteristics, there are still difficulties in using this type to correct any significant astigmatism as the lens moulds to the corneal shape. However, the newer types of soft lens that are now available seem to overcome this problem. Soft lenses are less durable than hard lenses and the need for more frequent replacement is an economic disadvantage. Some effort is being made to introduce disposable soft lenses which obviate the difficulties and nuisance of sterilization and so on.

Most soft lenses, like the hard ones, have to be removed daily, though there are some types available for prolonged wear. Constant wear is not yet achievable on any large scale, and it is customary to change—or at least remove—soft lenses, even the extended wear type, every two or three months.

The supply of contact lenses

Most contact lenses are supplied by optometrists, or ophthalmic opticians, following their assessment of the patient's requirements.

The fitting and ordering of contact lenses by an ophthalmologist is becoming more widespread. In fact, some ophthalmologists, particularly those well versed in corneal pathology, devote a major part of their professional activity to this. However, for most, it is not practical to do this because of the time required.

Problems with contact lenses

The problems experienced with contact lenses can be numerous, and mainly relate to the patient's inability to tolerate the lens on the eyeball, or to poor fitting. The posterior surface of the lens should follow closely the curvature of the cornea. The common complaint that there is 'a bit of grit under the lens' is usually not the case. The painful foreign body sensation is in fact arising from a minor corneal abrasion or erosion. The discomfort may be very unpleasant and sometimes presents itself several hours after the lens has been taken out, typically in the early hours of the morning. If the symptoms do not rapidly recede, and especially if the eye is significantly inflamed, medical referral to an eye department or eye casualty department may be necessary. The lens must not be inserted in the eye for several days or weeks; lens wear should then only be resumed gradually, otherwise the erosion of the cornea may recur. Fortunately permanent damage is rare, owing to the remarkable healing capacity of the cornea.

Other problems can arise from the variety of solutions used to store, clean, sterilize or remove protein from the lenses. Some are responsible for a chronic inflammation of the conjunctiva or cornea. Many of these solutions are unnecessarily complex, although there is no harm in patients who can tolerate them using them for convenience. However, hard Perspex lenses may be stored in tap water and soft lenses in saline prepared with sterilized water, without added preservatives. Of these, thiomesal, present in some proprietary preparations is now recognized as being particularly troublesome.

Magnifying glasses

In many cases, a disease of the eye causing defective vision can be helped with magnification, most notably senile macular degeneration. In other retinal conditions such as diabetic retinopathy (if not too advanced) and even in a moderate degree of cataract, a magnifying glass can be helpful for reading.

A hand magnifier is the simplest device, but if the patient has a physical handicap, such as arthritis or a tremor, which makes holding the glass difficult, a stand magnifier can be used or one that is held around the neck. Illumination may also be incorporated into the instruments.

Patients often ask why the same effect cannot be produced by 'increasing the power of the spectacles'. This is not possible, although complicated spectacle borne devices with increased

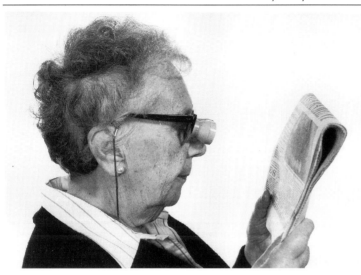

Figure 7.16   A more sophisticated visual aid of the telescopic type.

magnification are available, even telescopes (Figure 7.16).

Closed circuit television screen magnifiers are now available, but are very expensive. A promising development is the advent of enlarging copying machines, which can be of value in the scrutiny of particularly important documents or of music.

PRACTICAL POINTS

● Myopia, short-sightedness, causes blurred distance vision and is simply corrected by a concave lens.

● Hypermetropia is usually undetected if the individual has adequate accommodation for both distance as well as near vision. As this ability to accommodate begins to fail with age, the hypermetrope develops symptoms initially of blurred near vision, but eventually of distance vision too. The optical correction is by a convex lens.

● Everyone develops presbyopia in middle life. This requires the use of convex lenses for reading. If a distance correction is also required, two pairs of spectacles may be required. Alternatively both corrections may be incorporated in bifocal or varifocal spectacles.

● Anisometropia requires detection early in life to avoid the development of a lazy eye.

● Contact lenses are valuable cosmetically and optically, particularly for myopes. Problems of adaptation and tolerance mean they require more perseverance by the wearer and supervision by the supplier, than do spectacles.

8   The cornea and keratitis

The cornea

The cornea is part of the structural wall of the eyeball and is the first transparent optical medium through which light passes on its way to the retina.

The cornea owes its transparency, at least partially, to the regularity of the arrangement of its bundles of collagen, which are disposed in a laminar fashion; the direction of the bundles in one lamina is at right angles to that in the next. In the sclera, with which the cornea is contiguous, the collagen bundles are haphazardly arranged so that the sclera is translucent, not transparent. Any condition leading to a disruption of the regular geometrical relationship of the corneal collagen, such as destructive inflammation, may permanently reduce the cornea's transparency and impair the vision.

The collagen makes up the bulk of the corneal substance and is covered externally with a surface epithelium and lined internally with a layer of endothelial cells (Figure 8.1).

On both the inner and outer aspects, structureless layers separate the epithelium and endothelium from the substance. These cell layers keep the cornea at a low hydration. Failure of the endothelium, in particular, leads to oedema of the substance, again with some loss of vision owing to the disturbed transparency. The most serious cause of corneal oedema is a sudden rise in eye pressure, as in acute glaucoma, while the commonest cause is the overwearing of contact lenses.

The cornea is normally avascular and the only sensation it has is pain.

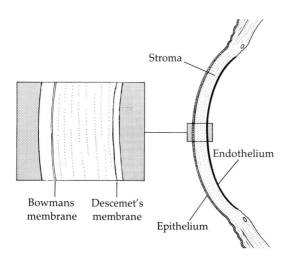

Figure 8.1 Structure of the cornea. The thickness is exaggerated. Normally the cornea is about 1 mm thick and slightly less in the axial region than in the periphery.

Keratitis

Superficial keratitis, an inflammation involving the surface, is the most common type of inflammation affecting the cornea. Deep keratitis occasionally arises as a primary condition, but is

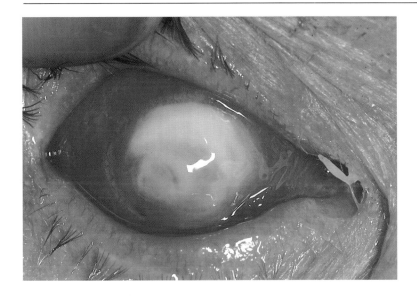

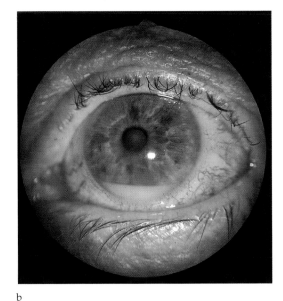

b

Figure 8.2 Two consequences of corneal ulceration: (*a*) a corneal abscess has resulted from severe pseudomonas infection; (*b*) a small central ulcer is associated with a hypopyon. A level of pus is seen in the anterior chamber.

usually a consequence of the superficial type. The condition is not considered in any detail here.

The symptoms which commonly result from superficial keratitis, a **corneal ulcer**, are those of a red eye, with injection mainly around the cornea, watering, irritability and a foreign body sensation. There may also be photophobia and some possible blurring of vision, depending on the situation of the ulcer.

Destruction of part of the epithelium is recognized clinically by fluorescein staining (see Chapter 3). The pupil of the eye is also either normal or slightly reduced in size. Primary corneal ulceration is commonly infective.

Infective corneal ulcers

Bacterial ulcers These may be of any severity. Ulcers caused by either the pneumococcus, or by pseudomonas (Figure 8.2a), are particularly important, both possibly being associated with pus in the anterior chamber—a hypopyon (Figure 8.2b).

Bacterial ulcers may also occur following injury or exposure of the eye. This secondary corneal ulceration is discussed on page 66.

Virus ulceration may take many forms. A dendritic ulcer is an important variety of viral ulcer due to herpes simplex (Figure 8.3). Patients with this condition may have a history of cold sores around the mouth or on the lips. Like cold sores, dendritic ulceration may be recurrent.

Herpes zoster may also affect the cornea in a number of ways, producing, for example, superficial erosions or ulcers, or deep patches of inflammation in the corneal substance. As with herpes simplex, recurrences may occur for long periods, even years after the initial episode.

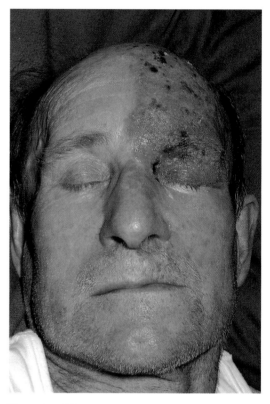

Figure 8.4 Herpes zoster ophthalmicus. Virtually the whole of the ophthalmic division of the trigeminal nerve is involved (see also Figure 17.18).

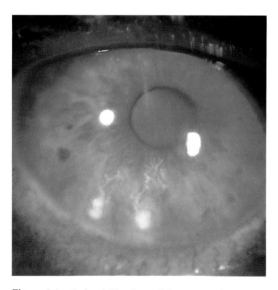

Figure 8.3 A dendritic ulcer of the cornea due to herpes simplex. Fluorescein staining of the cornea is often seen best in a blue light.

Herpes zoster can be particularly unpleasant in its propensity to leave a numb cornea, which, irrespective of recurrence, is at risk from unrecognized repeated minor traumata.

The full blown picture of herpes zoster is unmistakable (Figure 8.4). After a few days of severe pain in the region of the ophthalmic division of the trigeminal, vesicles appear on the skin in that area. The eye may be affected early or late, or both, or may sometimes appear to be unaffected until the active phase of the skin eruption is almost over. It has been said that the

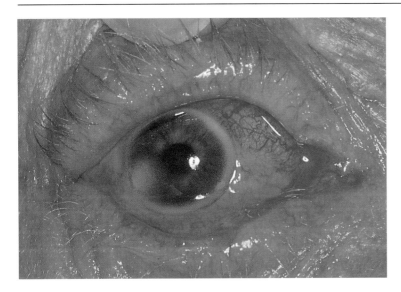

Figure 8.5 A marginal ulcer of the cornea.

eye is usually involved if vesicles appear on the side of the nose. Apart from keratitis, there may also be an associated iridocyclitis with pupillary dilatation due to iris destruction. Scleritis may also occur.

Superficial punctate keratitis may take the form of multiple tiny areas of epithelial loss, with or without subepithelial infiltration of the cornea. Even with fluorescein staining, these may be detectable only by slit-lamp examination. Herpes simplex, the adenoviruses and the chlamydia organisms may affect the cornea in this way.

Epithelial erosions of this type are a frequent and important complication, or association, of virus or chlamydial infections which may present initially as conjunctivitis (see Chapter 14). Perhaps the most important of these is trachoma,

where other serious corneal involvement can occur (see page 132).

Marginal ulcer

A marginal ulcer is a common, non-infective ulcer which is not normally severely disabling and is usually self-healing (Figure 8.5). As its name implies, the ulcer is situated close to the corneoscleral junction.

Other corneal ulcers

Other ulcers that can be recurrent are associated with skin conditions such as rosacea. Rosacea tends to occur particularly in the lower part of the cornea, and these ulcers may heal and leave the cornea scarred and thin (see Chapter 25).

Secondary corneal ulceration

Secondary corneal ulceration can be caused by a failure of ocular protection (see page 162). The predisposing conditions are:

1 Loss of corneal sensation from neurological causes, perhaps following Gasserian surgery for tic, or resulting from herpes zoster (see above).

2 Inability of the eyelids to close, as in Bell's palsy, or due to extreme protrusion of the eye as a result of dysthyroid disease.

3 Corneal drying, as in tear deficiency – Sjögren's syndrome – (see Chapter 15), or due to a combination of all the above factors.

Consequences of corneal ulceration

Many corneal ulcers heal with, and sometimes without, treatment, leaving no sequels. Not uncommonly, however, there may be scarring at the site of the ulceration.

Corneal opacity If the scarring is axial in the cornea, the vision of the eye may be permanently impaired. In these circumstances, some improvement in vision may be obtained with spectacles, but a contact lens may give better vision. In severe cases, a corneal graft will be required in order to improve the sight (Figure 8.6).

Perforation of the cornea The ultimate complication of an ulceration is perforation of the cornea, which may happen in spite of treatment. Several possible complications may result. For example, the iris may adhere to the cornea

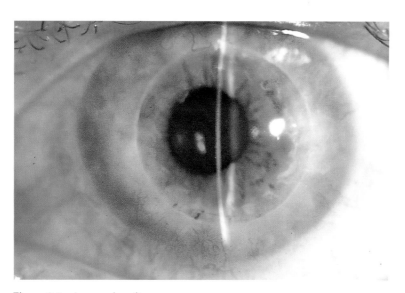

Figure 8.6 A corneal graft.

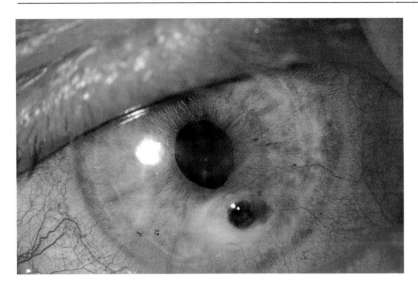

Figure 8.7 A perforation of the cornea with prolapse through it of the iris, which appears quite black.

(anterior synechia) or may actually prolapse through the hole (Figure 8.7); cataract may occur and glaucoma may result from the obliteration of the angle of the anterior chamber when the aqueous humour is lost. An added danger is an infection taking hold in the inner eye (endophthalmitis) with the possible loss of the eye as a useful organ.

Treatment of corneal ulcers

Treatment of corneal ulcers is directed to the cause. Local anti-infective agents, antibiotics or antivirals are used, as appropriate. In severe cases, systemic chemotherapy is necessary (see Chapter 21).

The eye should be kept padded and the pupil dilated with drops. Atropine (1 per cent) is used in severe cases, otherwise something weaker such as cyclopentolate (1 per cent) may be used.

Chemical cauterization is a time-honoured method of treatment of recalcitrant corneal ulcers. The eye is locally anaesthetized and phenol or iodine is applied to the affected area of the cornea, after removal of dead epithelium.

The use of local steroids may be dangerous because the effect can be to whiten the eye, while allowing the ulceration to run rampant. This is particularly the case with herpes simplex, the dendritic ulcer. Marginal or rosaceal ulcers may improve with steroids, but these drugs should be given only under an ophthalmologist's direct supervision. A slit-lamp examination is mandatory for monitoring the progress or adverse effect of the drugs.

Corneal degeneration

Corneal degenerations form a curious group of diseases which may be associated with a severe disturbance or loss of vision:

- Bullous keratopathy

- Hereditary corneal dystrophies

- Conical cornea

- Pterygium (a 'wing')

- Band-shaped degeneration

- Arcus senilis.

Bullous keratopathy

Bullous keratopathy may occur as a sequel to any of the conditions that give rise to corneal oedema, with associated blurring of vision. The 'bullae' are small fluid-containing vesicles in the epithelium which sometimes rupture and result in episodes of sharp pain. This condition is a feature found in eyes with severe uncontrolled glaucoma or disease of the endothelium, which fails to dehydrate the cornea. Such a disease may be primary, the so-called 'endothelial corneal dystrophy of Fuchs', or may follow damage to the endothelium during intraocular surgery, particularly cataract extraction and especially when an intraocular implant is introduced (Figure 8.8).

Hereditary corneal dystrophies

In these conditions, amazing diverse patterns of opacity occur and produce pretty slit-lamp appearances. The effect on the patient's vision varies; in some patients there is severe visual loss, while in others the sight is hardly affected.

Conical cornea

In this condition (keratoconus) the cornea is thinned at its apex and assumes a cone shape

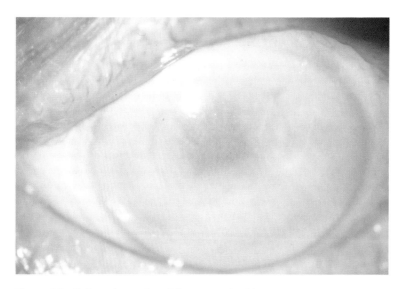

Figure 8.8 Bullous dystrophy of the cornea, in this case a consequence of cataract surgery with a now outdated type of lens implant.

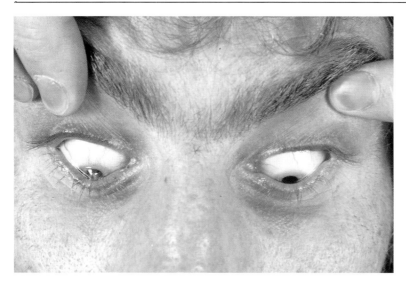

Figure 8.9 Conical cornea. The conical shape is often best appreciated by having the patient look down, when the tented appearance of the lower lid is emphasized, in this case on the right side.

(Figure 8.9). Ordinary spectacles are less helpful than contact lenses, though even these may be ineffective in some cases. It occurs most frequently in young men but it also found in some subjects with atopic eczema or with Down's syndrome.

If the sight does not improve sufficiently with contact lenses or spectacles then, as with other corneal dystrophies and bullous keratopathy, corneal grafting may have to be considered.

Historically, corneal grafting is one of the oldest forms of transplantation. Apart from technical considerations, the success of this operation is aided by the avascularity of the cornea which presumably prevents blood-borne factors, likely to lead to rejection, from reaching the graft.

Pterygium (a 'wing')

This common condition is found in people living in hot climates. It presents as a wing-shaped overgrowth of conjunctival tissues, characteristically covering the nasal margin of the cornea (Figure 8.10). They do have some cosmetic disadvantage, but it is rare for such a lesion to extend to the axial cornea where it would, of course, lead to loss of sight. Nevertheless, a progressive overgrowth should prompt surgical removal.

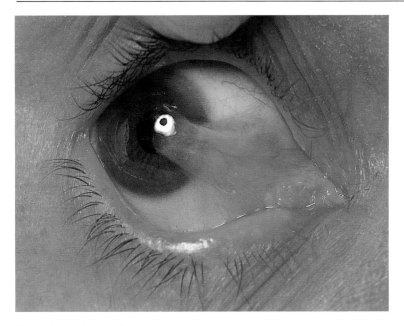

Figure 8.10   A pterygium.

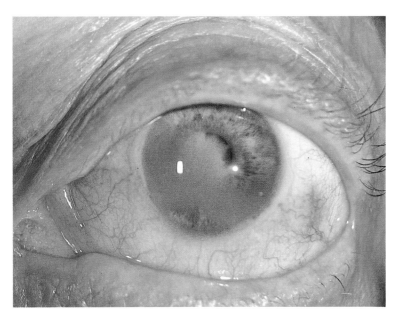

Figure 8.11   Band-shaped degeneration of the cornea:
the typical calcified appearance.

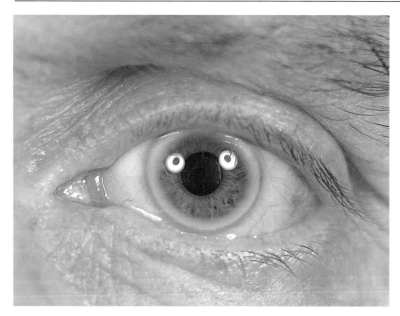

Figure 8.12   Arcus senilis.

Band-shaped degeneration

This condition is due to the deposition of calcium in the superficial corneal layers (Figure 8.11). It occures in diverse circumstances. Occasionally it is a primary condition; sometimes it is associated with hypercalcaemia. It is also found in cases of long-standing uveitis (see Still's disease, Chapter 25) and is often noted in blind, degenerate eyes.

If treatment is indicated because of painful flaking of calcium or because the sight is affected, the calcium can be scraped off, perhaps with the use of the chelating agent, disodium versenate. Very occasionally, corneal grafting is needed.

Arcus senilis

The greyish-white ring of arcus senilis is found close to but slightly separated from the limbus (the corneoscleral junction) (Figure 8.12). The condition is a common feature present in middle and old age.

Arcus senilis has no effect on vision and is only occasionally severe enough to be thought of as a cosmetic blemish. Although a lipid deposit, its relationship to raised serum cholesterol, and by implication to atheromatous arterial disease of the heart (or elsewhere), is unproven. Its appearance in early adult life may raise suspicions in that direction, however.

PRACTICAL POINTS

● The cornea is normally transparent and any disturbance may therefore blur vision.

● Inflammation of the cornea is frequently infective in origin. It often affects the surface, producing a corneal ulcer which is a common cause of the acute red eye.

● Secondary corneal ulcers occur through failure of ocular protection.

● Perforation of the cornea is the ultimate complication of ulceration, but short of this a corneal ulcer may produce scarring which seriously damages the vision.

● Degenerative diseases of the cornea may result in severe disturbance or loss of vision.

9   Uveitis: iridocyclitis and choroiditis

The uvea is the collective term used for the iris, ciliary body and the choroid (Figure 9.1). It is the intermediate vegetative functional layer of the eye between its structural coat (sclera behind, cornea in front) and the light sensitive layer, the retina.

● The iris is opaque and acts as the shutter of the eye by adjusting the size of the pupil, its central aperture.

● The ciliary body produces aqueous humour, and encloses the ciliary muscle, contraction of

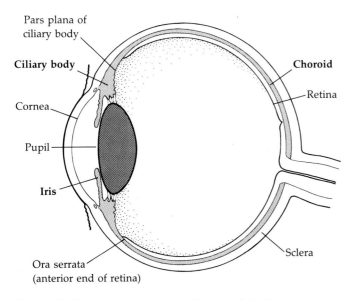

Pars plana of ciliary body

Ciliary body

Cornea

Pupil

Iris

Ora serrata
(anterior end of retina)

Choroid

Retina

Sclera

Figure 9.1   The structures of the uveal tract are in bold type.

which allows the lens to accommodate, thus altering the focus of the eyes.

● The choroid is a nutritional layer to the retina, as well as acting as a pigment layer to prevent internal scattering of the light.

Although congenital anomalies, tumours and degenerative disease occur in uveal tissue, the commonest pathology is inflammation, uveitis.

Oddly, in uveitis, the conventional causes of inflammation are hardly ever found to exist. Though uveitis is a common condition, direct infections are rare, being mostly a sequel to trauma.

Types of uveitis

Uveal inflammation can simultaneously involve the iris, ciliary body and the choroid, the condition being termed a panuveitis. More frequently, however, the condition involves only the anterior uvea, the iris (iritis) and the ciliary body (cyclitis).

Anterior uveitis: iritis and iridocyclitis

Inflammation of the iris and ciliary body usually presents as an acute and possibly painful, often photophobic, red eye with blurred vision and injection characteristically around the corneoscleral junction.

● The pupil tends to be small, or at least reluctant to dilate, and may be irregular because the exudation into the anterior chamber 'sticks' the pupil margin to the lens. These adhesions are known as 'posterior synechiae' (Figure 9.2).

● Positive diagnosis of anterior uveitis can be made only by a slit-lamp examination. The signs include flare (a Tyndall effect) and cells in the aqueous humour, and keratic precipitates (kp) on the back of the cornea. These are punctate collections of inflammatory cells (Figure 9.3).

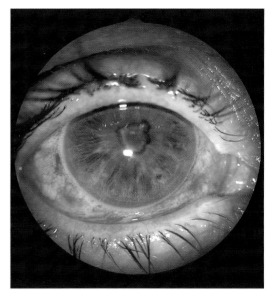

Figure 9.2   An irregular pupil in a case of iritis. The pupil itself is filled with exudate; the iris is bound down to the lens by adhesions–posterior synechiae.

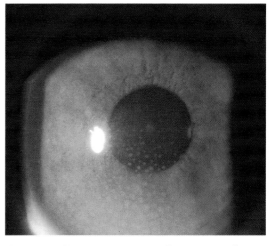

Figure 9.3   Keratic precipitates. These are usually visible only by slit-lamp examination.

If a slit-lamp is unavailable, the non-specialist may have difficulty in distinguishing a mild anterior uveitis from a conjunctivitis, as both the vision and the pupil may be normal. In a case of iritis, for example, there is no discharge and the injection of the eye tends to be around the cornea.

It is excusable to treat a mild case of iritis with antibiotics, as if it were conjunctivitis. This at least does no harm as long as the patient is monitored. If the condition fails to improve, however, the patient should be sent to a specialist.

Posterior uveitis — choroiditis

Inflammation of the choroid alone usually occurs without any external sign; the eyes do not become red.

Symptoms may arise from the effect on the overlying retina. Choroiditis may have a damaging effect on the vision if the affected area underlies, or is close to, the macula. The condition can lead to permanent loss of central vision if treatment is delayed or ineffective. Other symptoms result from the exudates which enter the vitreous cavity via the retina. The patient will complain of spots in the vision or, if the exudate is severe, the sight will be obscured. Similar complaints may arise from inflammation of the most posterior part of the ciliary body which faces the vitreous.

Such vitreous opacities are readily seen with the ophthalmoscope and have to be distinguished from other causes of floaters or spots in the vision. A search should be made for a focus of acute choroiditis; with the ophthalmoscope this appears as a fuzzy-edged white area which is actually retinal oedema (Figure 9.4). The view is hazy, interfered with as it is by the vitreous exudate. When the inflammation subsides, clumps of pigment released from the cells of the choroid make a characteristic feature surrounding white areas which, at the burnt out stage, are simply sclera seen through destroyed areas of retina or choroid (Figure 9.5).

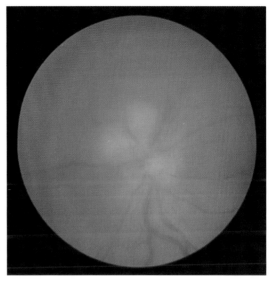

Figure 9.4 Acute choroiditis in its active phase. Two white patches are seen above the optic disc. The view is hazy owing to inflammatory exudate in the vitreous.

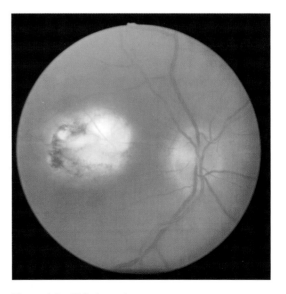

Figure 9.5 Old choroiditis.

Causes of uveitis

Large texts on ophthalmology may list about a hundred associations of uveitis. Unfortunately, in most cases, extensive investigation will reveal nothing.

The main related diseases are:

● **Ankylosing spondylitis** associated with iridocyclitis; the latter is especially found in young men. Ankylosing spondylitis has an association with the possession of the HLA B_{27} factor, and is often familial.

● **Sarcoidosis** causes a more chronic type of iridocyclitis.

● **Toxoplasmosis** causes choroiditis in both adults and children. Intra-uterine infection with toxoplasmosis may lead to infantile choroiditis, which may be undiscovered until later in life, unless the infection produces widespread systemic effects.

● **Collagen diseases** All the collagen diseases may be associated with anterior uveitis and, in children, Still's disease is often unfortunately accompanied by severe, chronic uveitis.

Other odd forms of uveitis occur in Reiter's disease and, traditionally, in tuberculosis and syphilis, though these are comparatively rare. However, there is a definite association with Behçet's syndrome of orogenital ulceration.

Uveitis is also a feature of two important tropical diseases, leprosy and onchoceriasis.

In addition to these, two particular conditions need special mention: heterochromic cyclitis and sympathetic uveitis.

Heterochromic cyclitis

This is a strange, dormant, chronic anterior uveitis in which the iris becomes depigmented so that a brown eye becomes blue. The eye never becomes red, keratic precipitates are prominent, and unpigmented and posterior synechiae do not occur (Figure 9.6).

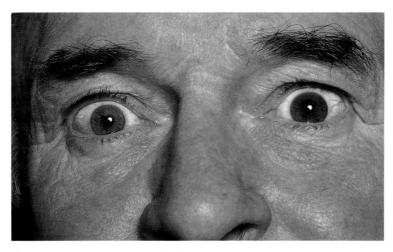

Figure 9.6 Heterochromic cyclitis showing depigmentation of the iris of the affected right eye.

The condition is also strictly unilateral and, after some years, cataract and glaucoma may occur.

Sympathetic uveitis

The condition occurs in cases of penetrating injury, especially when the ciliary body and lens are damaged. A few days, or weeks, after the injury a severe uveitis arises in the injured eye, followed shortly by a similar inflammation in the fellow eye. Sympathetic uveitis is considered in more detail in Chapter 18.

It should be noted that any ocular injury, whether a significant concussion or a penetrating wound directly involving the lens or uveal tissue, may lead to iridocyclitis of the injured eye. Perhaps the commonest and fortunately normally transient form of this occurs after surgery on the anterior segment of the eye; for example, after cataract extraction of all types, but especially when combined with lens implantation (see Chapter 10).

Investigation of uveitis

As mentioned, the investigation of uveitis is often fruitless, although it is customary to x-ray the chest and sacroiliac joints, and carry out a full blood count and erythrocyte sedimentation rate (ESR).

A Mantoux test may be helpful, mainly to confirm the expected negative result rather than to discover a tuberculous aetiology. A Kveim test for sarcoidosis may be advisable if the Mantoux is negative.

A general medical check-up is indicated, and glycosuria should be sought because diabetics are prone to uveitis. An autoimmune pathology should be looked for by examining the antinuclear factor. Serology is usually carried out for syphilis and gonorrhoea, and particularly for toxoplasmosis. If appropriate, a test for HLA B_{27} should also be performed.

Focal sepsis in the ear, nose and throat, the teeth or the sinuses, as well as in the bowel and urine, was once regarded as important in the aetiology of uveitis. However, the search for these sources if often futile and, if found, the treatment of them has never been convincingly related to the eradication of uveitis.

Treatment of uveitis

It would be useful to say that we treat the cause of uveitis, but as we have seen, in most cases one is never found. The standard treatment is the use of the steroid group of drugs given locally as drops in anterior uveitis and systemically for posterior uveitis, particularly when, in the latter case, the macula is threatened.

The steroid drops used for anterior uveitis are prednisolone, betamethasone and dexamethasone. These should be given frequently, even hourly. If not rapidly effective, there may be a need to supplement this with a subconjunctival injection or by systemic administration.

If the pupil is becoming bound down by posterior synechiae, drops to dilate it must be given; usually atropine (1 per cent), but in mild cases the weaker cyclopentolate (1 per cent) may be sufficient. Phenylephrine (10 per cent) drops may also be needed.

Toxoplasmosis may be helped by a course of pyrimethamine or spiramycin, to which the infective protozoan is usually sensitive; the effect of pyrimethamine is believed to be enhanced by giving sulphapyrimidine simultaneously. Frequent monitoring of the red and white blood count is advisable when pyrimethamine is given.

Complications of uveitis

Successful treatment of a particular attack of uveitis is unfortunately no guarantee against subsequent attacks. Furthermore, some cases of uveitis do not present in an acute form and are from the outset either less severe or chronic in character.

It is uncommon for an eye with uveitis to resist treatment but unfortunately this occasionally happens. Such an eye may eventually go completely blind and shrink, as the aqueous humour is no longer produced by the (destroyed) ciliary body, and the retina degenerates. This is the state known as phthisis bulbi.

In most cases of anterior uveitis, however, the clinical course is rapidly controlled by steroid drops, but in some cases complications arise which are usually found when the condition first presents.

Complications include:

- Glaucoma
- Cataract
- Macular oedema
- Vasculitis.

Glaucoma

Glaucoma may arise as a secondary condition to iridocyclitis and be due to embarrassment to the outflow of the fibrin-laden aqueous humour. Rarely, glaucoma may be caused by a complete blockage of the pupil by synechiae and exudate, leading to a damming up of the aqueous behind the distended iris (iris bombé). During this phase, the eye may be severely painful.

Once the pupil is dilated, and steroids quieten the inflammation, the secondary glaucoma subsides. Acetazolamide (250 mg, up to four times daily), given orally, may be needed to help tide the eye over the period of raised pressure. It should also be remembered that, in some patients with uveitis, the prolonged local use of steroids may itself cause a rise in eye pressure.

Cataract

A cataract may occur following a prolonged chronic anterior uveitis, with the vision of the eye slowly deteriorating. In some cases the cataract is simply the result of organized inflammatory debris over the pupillary area of the lens. In other cases, a true complicated cataract develops.

If the vision becomes severely affected, particularly if this involves both eyes, surgery may be necessary. Heterochromic cyclitis is particularly likely to lead to cataract.

Cataracts are discussed in more detail in Chapter 10.

Macular oedema

Macular oedema with disturbance or loss of central vision may complicate uveitis, either anterior or posterior.

Vasculitis

Vasculitis of the retinal vessels may be associated with uveitis, especially that due to sarcoidosis and other collagen diseases.

PRACTICAL POINTS

● Inflammation is the commonest disease of the uvea, usually involving either only the anterior uvea, the iris and the ciliary body or just the choroid.

● Without the benefit of a slit-lamp examination, it may be difficult to distinguish mild anterior uveitis from conjunctivitis. Particular attention should be paid to the state of the vision and of the pupil, which may be irregular and small.

● Posterior uveitis, choroiditis, may affect vision if it involves the central retina.

● To distinguish choroiditis from other causes of spots or floaters, an examination with the ophthalmoscope must be made for a characteristic fuzzy white area in the fundus.

● The causal link between uveitis and other diseases is tenuous. It is nevertheless customary, though often futile, to carry out investigations including x-rays, blood counts and ESR. Particular associations include ankylosing spondylitis, sarcoidosis, toxoplasmosis and, in children, Still's disease.

● The only treatment available at present is with steroids and these do not prevent subsequent attacks of uveitis. The pupil should be dilated by instilling mydriatic drops if there is any sign that its margin is becoming adherent to the lens.

● Complications of uveitis are glaucoma, cataract, macular oedema and vasculitis.

10   Cataracts

Cataract is a disturbance of the transparency of the lens of the eye. The lens acts as part of the focusing mechanism and is situated symmetrically across and in a plane perpendicular to the optical axis of the eye. It is held in this position by the zonule, or suspensory ligament, a curious sheet of fibrillar tissue which stretches from the ciliary body to the equatorial region of the lens. The shape of the lens is altered in accommodation. In this function the ciliary muscle contracts, narrowing the ring attachment of the zonule. The tension of this on the lens relaxes, and the lens then bulges on account of the intrinsic elasticity of its capsule. The increased convexity of the lens provides for clear focusing of near objects.

Within its capsule the lens substance is roughly divisible into a central harder nucleus, surrounded by a softer cortical zone (Figure 10.1). In the very young the nucleus is small, but enlarges with the growth of the lens, the latter proceeding throughout life.

Any opacity in the lens of the eye is the condition termed cataract. While many types of opacity may occur, the most important is cataract occurring in old age, senile cataract. Before discussing senile cataract in greater detail, two important points should be noted:

1 Cataracts may be discovered at any age. Indeed important forms of cataracts may be congenital or inherited.

2 The effect of lens opacity (a less emotive term for cataract) on the patient's vision depends on how severely the lens is affected and what part has lost its clarity.

The position of the opacity in relation to the 'front to the back axis' (the optic axis) is of particular importance. For example, if the opacity is positioned so that light passing through the

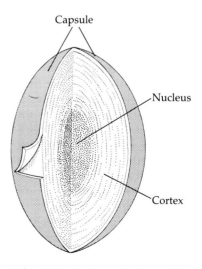

Figure 10.1 A schematic view of the lens of the eye.

pupil towards the macula is obstructed, a marked disability may result, even if the opacity is small.

Alternatively a small and perhaps non-progressive opacity, tucked away behind the iris, may have no effect on the patient's sight; here it is pointless to inform (and thus alarm) the patient that 'a cataract is forming' because the future progression of a lens opacity of any type is not always predictable.

Many types, though not all, of developmental opacities are stationary. Even senile cataract (usually progressive) may progress slowly or sometimes not at all.

Recognizing cataract

When the lens is totally opacified, the pupil appears white (Figure 10.2), indicating a mature cataract. At this stage no red reflex is obtained on looking into the eye with an ophthalmoscope.

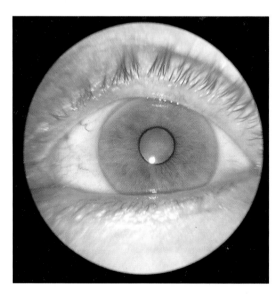

Figure 10.2 The white pupil in a case of mature cataract.

If the cataract is not well-advanced, fragments of red reflex may be seen, interrupted by the black shadows of the lens opacity. The shadows are often of a characteristic shape and indicate the type of cataract present (see below).

Any degree of cataract may make it difficult to see the retina, but with a very early cataract, if the pupil is dilated with drops, it is often possible to examine the retina fully to ensure there are no defects present. It is essential to ascertain that everything in the posterior segment is normal because, if the cataract advances, this view will be impossible. It is important to know in advance that the improvement in vision after surgery will not be hindered by an unsuspected macular or other retinal defect.

Senile cataract

Senile cataract is an important type of opacity, indeed it is the most important eye disease occurring in old age. If the lens opacifies to any extent, the vision becomes blurred and eventually very poor indeed (Figures 10.3–10.6).

The condition is of unknown aetiology, commonly occurring in patients over the age of seventy years. Opacities of a similar type can often occur earlier, though rarely before the age of fifty years, with the following results:

● Sight is blurred, usually more in one than the other eye. In the early stages, sight may be improved with a change of spectacles, especially as a degree of myopia often develops as an accompaniment to the onset of cataract. Paradoxically this myopia may, in a few cases, actually help the reading vision, even without spectacles, for some time before the opacity becomes dense.

● In most patients, reading is particularly irksome owing to the associated smallness of the pupil, obscuring a proportion of the available clear lens. For this reason some patients with early cataract are particularly troubled by bright sunlight.

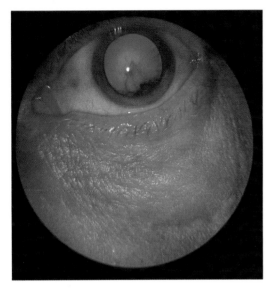

Figure 10.3   The view with the ophthalmoscope in a case of early cortical cataract.

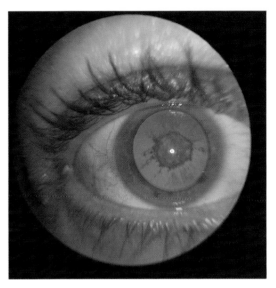

Figure 10.4   A similar view of posterior cortical cataract.

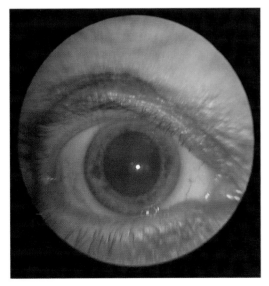

Figure 10.5   The ophthalmoscopic view in a case of advanced cataract. Only a faint red reflex remains.

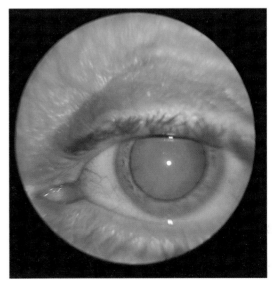

Figure 10.6   The ophthalmoscopic view of early nuclear cataract.

• Dazzle and glare from oncoming headlights at night are frequent complaints by patients even with minor lens opacities.

• A steady deterioration occurs in the majority of cases. Eventually the whole lens may opacify and the patient's vision is reduced. Although light can be seen, the eye becomes effectively blind. Naturally this is particularly distressing for the patient if the condition is advanced in both eyes.

Management of senile cataract

If an early lens opacity is discovered during a routine sight test for spectacles, no special action is necessary as long as the patient has no complaints and if, with suitable optical correction, the vision is improved to a satisfactory level. It is at least arguable that there is little point in upsetting the patient by telling him or her of the discovery until a subsequent examination shows that the condition is progressive in nature. In any event, at this early stage, there are no medical measures, pills or drops, that will arrest or reverse the progress of the cataract.

If the patient complains of blurred vision, the first therapeutic step is a new optical correction, perhaps tinted if the opacities are positioned axially. It is as well to remember that an elderly person's reading vision is just as important as clear distance vision, if not more so. It is worth advising the patient to read with a good light of optimal rather than maximal brightness, directed from behind the shoulder on to the page. A simple magnifier may also be useful. To reduce the glare from the page, a piece of dark card the width of the page with a horizontal slit cut into it can be helpful.

Surgical measures

There is no firm ruling as to when surgery should be considered for senile cataract. However, generally, the opinion is that this should be undertaken when the visual impairment seriously hampers the individual's quality of life. Modern cataract surgery is largely successful with cataracts at almost any stage of development, so the historical criterion of the 'maturity' of the cataract, or 'waiting until it gets ripe', is no longer relevant.

As a benchmark, surgery is usually considered when the vision of the less affected eye falls to about 6/18 or 20/60 (four lines on the distance chart) or N.8 for reading.

Techniques of cataract surgery

The techniques of modern cataract surgery are too numerous and complex to detail here, but two important principles should help in guiding the choice of method:

1 Cataract surgery involves the removal from the eye of all or a substantial part of the opaque lens.

2 In an elderly patient, the way in which cataract surgery is undertaken will depend very much on the physical hardness of the centre of the lens, the nucleus. As noted, this occurs because the nucleus and hence lens itself grows throughout life by adding on layers of new material from its equator.

Removal of the lens nucleus is the key stage in the management of senile cataract and the classical procedures for doing this are intracapsular and extracapsular cataract extraction.

Intracapsular cataract extraction   In this operation an incision is made in the eye, through which the whole lens is taken out. The nucleus is removed within the capsule of the lens, the latter containing both cortex and nucleus. In this procedure the zonular ligament which attaches the lens to the ciliary body is broken, or dissolved, by instilling the enzyme alpha-chymotrypsin for one or two minutes, and the lens extracted by a cryoprobe. The wound in the eye is then sutured (Figure 10.7).

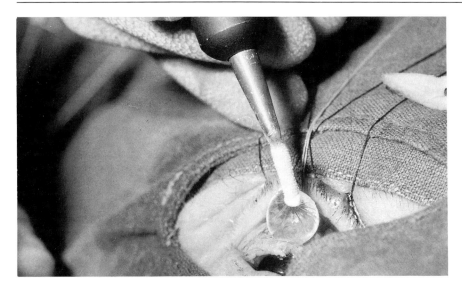

Figure 10.7   Removal of the entire lens using the
cryoprobe in the operation of intracapsular cataract
extraction.

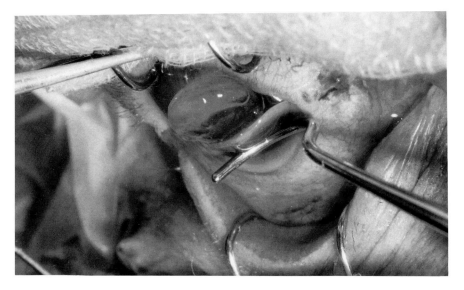

Figure 10.8   Removal of the lens nucleus during the
operation of extracapsular cataract extraction.

Extracapsular cataract extraction This older method has recently returned to popularity. A slightly smaller incision than that for the intracapsular method is made. A portion of the anterior segment of the capsule of the lens is removed, capsulectomy, and the nucleus is taken out through the wound (Figure 10.8). The cortical lens matter is either irrigated or sucked out of the eye. The technique leaves the posterior capsule intact, but in many cases this offers no significant obstruction to vision. In some instances a further minor operation, posterior capsulotomy, may be necessary to make a gap in this membrane. This procedure may be performed at the time of the original surgery. Alternatively it is done later, and a YAG laser may be used for this purpose.

Ultrasound The nucleus may be 'mashed up' using high frequency pulsating energy (ultrasound) to fragment the material, which is then irrigated and aspirated out of the eye. This can be achieved via an incision smaller than that used for formal cataract surgery. The technique, known as phaco-emulsification, though neat and effective, requires elaborate apparatus, but for the patient the small incision means a confident and early discharge from hospital, or the whole procedure even being carried out on an outpatient basis.

Optical problems after cataract surgery

The optical problems of an eye from which the lens has been removed are considerable. Essentially the eye becomes very hypermetropic and, in order for it to focus a clear image on the retina, a powerful convex spectacles lens must be worn. In an elderly patient previously blinded by bilateral senile cataract, surgery followed by prescription of such spectacles is still the classical management. There are, however, some considerable disadvantages to wearing the thick, heavy cataract 'pebble' spectacles:

● Everything looks large, so that the patient has difficult judging distances correctly, especially when walking about.

● The thickness of the lenses produces a distorted view when the patient looks through them at an oblique angle.

● The enlarged view from the operated, or aphakic, eye is a particular problem when a cataract is predominately or entirely one-sided. A cataract spectacle lens simply cannot be worn in the hope that the two eyes will cooperate. The images from the two eyes are of different sizes and cannot be fused into one. If an attempt is made to do so the result will be intolerable double vision. There are two answers to this problem:

1 Following conventional surgery, a contact lens may be used. This will not magnify the vision as much as a cataract spectacle lens.

2 An intraocular lens may be implanted during the original cataract surgery. The technique is now widely practised. The lens is sited in front of the iris, in the plane of the pupil, or behind the iris, the latter being the more favoured position to date (Figures 10.9–10.11). The resurgence of interest in the extracapsular technique is partly due to the development of implantation, the intact posterior lens capsule supporting the implant inserted behind the iris, or the implant itself being placed within the capsular 'bag'.

It is also possible to introduce implants some time after 'classical' cataract surgery (this is known as secondary implantation), should the wearing of a spectacle correction or contact lens be intolerable.

The implantation of an intraocular lens results in the retinal image size being virtually normal, allowing binocular vision to be restored by surgery carried out at an early stage in the cataract's development. The prediction of the required optical power for an implanted lens is still uncertain, but is greatly helped by ultrasonic measurement of the length of the eye, an

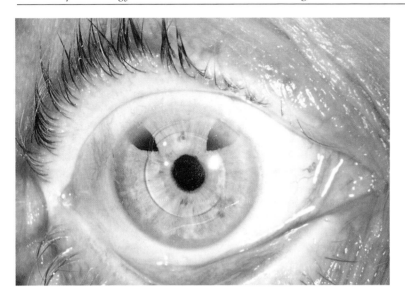

Figure 10.9 An anterior chamber lens implant.

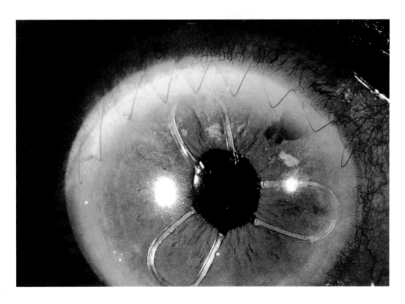

Figure 10.10 A pupil-supported implant of the
Severin type.

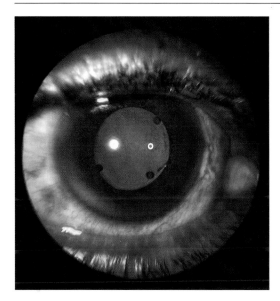

Figure 10.11 A posterior chamber implant. Dialling holes can be seen and, *bottom right*, part of one of the two loops which supports the lens behind the iris.

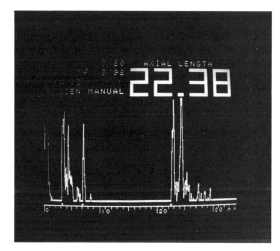

Figure 10.12 The ultrasonic picture obtained by the A-scan technique. The spikes represent, *left* to *right*, the cornea, both surfaces of the lens and the retina. The superimposed scale below indicates how the axial length of the eye can be measured.

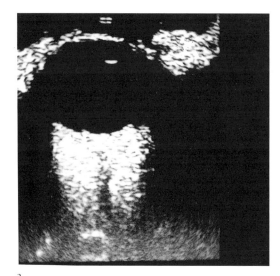

a

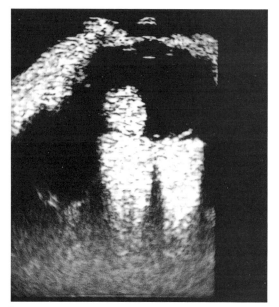

b

Figure 10.13 (*a*) The ultrasonic picture of the eye obtained by the B-scan technique. Echoes representing the front and back surfaces of the cornea and of the lens as well as of the concave surface of the retina are visible. (*b*) A B-scan which shows a large abnormal series of echoes from a malignant melanoma of the choroid.

important factor in its optical state, by the A-scan technique (Figure 10.12).

A slightly different, and valuable, ultrasound technique produces the so-called B-scan, a picture of the back of the eye when opacity of the media, for example a dense cataract, precludes any view of the integrity of the structures behind the lens. The scan could indicate that a retinal detachment was present, or perhaps some other condition that might equally contraindicate cataract surgery (Figure 10.13).

The long-term effect of intraocular lens implants is unknown, partly because frequent changes of technique and design do not permit adequate follow-up investigation. Some surgeons have lingering doubts about the long-term results of implantation and avoid its use in cataract surgery on 'only' eyes, where binocularity does not need to be considered.

General complications of cataract surgery

All forms of cataract surgery, with or without intraocular lens implantation, may be followed by complications.

Iritis Some degree of uveitis is almost inevitable after cataract surgery and prompts the prophylactic and therapeutic use of local steroid drops.

True pyogenic infection is a very serious but uncommon sequel and requires vigorous local and systemic chemotherapy.

Glaucoma This may take several forms and may occur in the very early postoperative period, usually temporarily. Late glaucoma is a sequel to defective healing of the cataract incision, the anterior chamber of the eye failing to reform as rapidly as it should.

Retinal detachment Patients who have had cataract surgery have an increased liability to develop retinal detachments. This is not usually an early event and may occur even years after the cataract surgery has been performed. Some believe that this complication is less likely to occur after extracapsular than after intracapsular extraction.

There are two complications that are more likely after intraocular implant surgery than after conventional cataract surgery. These are, first, corneal decompensation, the inability to keep the cornea 'dehydrated' (see Chapter 8), thus leading to bullous dystrophy and, second, cystoid oedema of the macula. There are several possible causes for each of these conditions.

● **Bullous dystrophy** results, at least to some extent, from mechanical damage (perhaps inevitable) to the corneal endothelium during implantation. Many surgeons consider a patient with a pre-existing corneal endothelial disease as being unsuitable for implantation. Bullous keratopathy, if it occurs, seriously reduces the vision and may be an indication for corneal grafting (see Figure 8.8).

● **Oedema of the macula** may be induced by prostaglandins being released from the iris and seeping back to the retina. Bright operating theatre lights focused on to the macula, via the implant, during surgery have also been incriminated. This is certainly an unfortunate sequel to implant surgery. The condition may arise some months after the procedure, when previously good postoperative vision suddenly becomes worse. The condition is often unresponsive to any treatment, but spontaneous improvement occurs in some cases.

Other forms of cataract

There are a number of different forms of cataract which may be classified as follows:

● Congenital cataract

● Cataract and general disease

● Traumatic cataract.

Congenital cataract

Some types of cataract are familial in origin, classically the 'zonular' or 'lamellar' cataract where a shell of opacity develops, surrounding and surrounded by clear lens substance.

An important type of cataract is associated with maternal rubella; unfortunately the condition is sometimes associated with a degenerative choroido-retinitis. Numerous varieties of cataract also occur in association with congenital errors of metabolism and chromosomal abnormalities, as in Down's syndrome.

If the cataract is bilateral, severe and present in early life, nystagmus will develop. Early surgery is indicated. As noted, the nucleus of the lens in the very young is virtually non-existent so the soft cataractous material can simply be washed or aspirated out of the eye.

A uniocular congenital cataract should not be treated with a view to restoring vision. Surgical attempts to do this invariably fail. The cause of the failure is amblyopia, the lazy eye (see Chapter 19), which prevents any improvement in sight, even following technically the most successful surgery to remove the opacity. If the eye is unsightly, cosmetic measures are all that are indicated for the associated squint or white pupil.

Cataract and general disease

Every patient discovered to have a lens opacity should have a urinanalysis to investigate the possibility of glycosuria, as diabetics are particularly likely to develop cataract.

In an elderly patient, a diabetic cataract appears as a variant of senile cataract. In the young, unstable diabetic a rapidly progressing opacification of the lens may occur.

Toxic factors also play a part in some lens opacities. For example, the prolonged use of systemic steroids is an important factor; rheumatoid patients are particularly susceptible. For the same reason patients who are immunosuppressed after transplantation may develop this so-called 'steroid cataract'.

Less common associations of cataract include myotonic dystrophy, skin atopy and hypocalcaemia.

Traumatic cataract

The condition may occur as a result of a blunt or penetrating trauma to the eye. Localized and stationary opacities sometimes result from concussion injuries, and the lens may become displaced or dislocated.

Penetration of the lens by glass fragments, or other foreign bodies, often leads to opacification of the whole lens. The lens injury is commonly part of more complex damage involving the cornea, sclera or the uveal tract. Penetrating injuries involving the lens are likely to lead to uveitis (see Chapter 18), occasionally of the

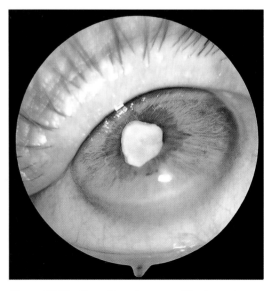

Figure 10.14 Complicated cataract. The irregular, bound-down pupil indicates previous uveitis in the eye.

sympathetic variety, though this is extremely rare.

Another less common sequel to an eye injury is dislocation of the lens (see page 176), which is particularly prone to become cataractous. Dislocation is not always traumatic; it may occur congenitally, as in Marfan's syndrome, of which the other most notable features are long extremities (arachnodactyly: spider fingers) and disease of the wall of the major arteries such as the aorta.

Radiation injury to the lens may lead to cataract, often with a latent period after exposure of some years. The prognosis for surgery for a radiation cataract, if indicated by the patient's vision, is not necessarily dismal, provided the general health is no contraindication.

Complicated cataract

The term 'complicated cataract' is used to describe any lens opacity which occurs as a result of some other disease of the eye. Longstanding uveitis (Figure 10.14), an untreated retinal detachment or an intraocular tumour are all examples of an associated disease; traumatic cataract is sometimes included in this category (see page 176).

PRACTICAL POINTS

● The most important type of cataract, being by far the most common, is senile cataract.

● The adequacy or otherwise of the patient's vision for the visual tasks required is the determining factor in deciding whether to operate on the cataract.

● The most successful outcome of surgery for senile cataract is achieved with the implantation of an intraocular lens, although the long-term effects have not yet been fully assessed.

● Complications of cataract surgery are iritis, glaucoma and retinal detachment.

● Rarer complications of cataract surgery include bullous keratopathy and oedema of the macula, but these are particular complications of procedures including lens implantation.

● Severe bilateral congenital cataract is an indication for surgery very early in life. However early this is undertaken, nystagmus often develops.

● Uniocular congenital cataract is best left untreated. Little visual improvement is obtained by removing it as the eye is amblyopic.

11   The vitreous humour

The vitreous fills the space behind the lens, between the lens and retina. It has a slightly gelatinous structure, with a yellowish tinge, and is transparent like the other ocular media, the cornea, aqueous humour and lens. The gel has a protein fibrillar matrix within it, but through the interstices of the matrix there is only a very slow percolation of fluid. Therefore, when any foreign material enters the vitreous, it tends to stay there for a long time, even though it may be mobile within the gel.

The boundary of the vitreous posteriorly is in contact with the retina, but is actually attached to the optic disc. Peripherally the vitreous adheres to the anterior part of the retina and ciliary body.

Symptoms and signs of vitreous disturbance

The symptoms of a mild vitreous disturbance are spots in the vision and shadows that may intermittently blur the sight, and 'floaters' which may in some circumstances be described as a recognizable object such as a fly.

The characteristic clinical sign of vitreous disturbance is the appearance of mobile black particles seen against the red reflex with the ophthalmoscope.

More severe involvement of the vitreous may lead to such an extensive opacification that the sight is not merely intermittently obscured but substantially and constantly impaired, sometimes to the point of effective blindness. Associated with this, the red reflex usually obtained with the ophthalmoscope may be completely obliterated.

The main conditions affecting the vitreous are degenerative changes, inflammation leading to debris in the vitreous and vitreous haemorrhage.

The differential diagnosis of the conditions is sometimes difficult to reach without a specialist examination. However, only inflammation and haemorrhage obscure to any serious degree the red reflex from the fundus.

● Inflammatory changes can usually be diagnosed with certainty either by catching a glimpse through the 'murk' of a white area of the retina, indicating choroiditis, or by a slit-lamp examination showing the presence of inflammatory cells in the anterior chamber of the eye, as well as behind the lens.

● Haemorrhage may require a slit-lamp examination to identify the opacities in the vitreous as red blood cells. It is easy for the non-specialist to misinterpret an absent red reflex produced by a vitreous haemorrhage as an advanced cataract. The history of the onset is likely to be of some help in the diagnosis, as the loss of vision from a cataract is unlikely to be acute.

In lesser degrees of haemorrhage, where some view of the retina can be obtained, the diagnosis is suggested by the finding of one or more retinal haemorrhages, for example, in a diabetic with the presence of new vessels (see page 223).

The cause of vitreous disturbance

Degenerative changes

Degenerative changes in the vitreous may take may forms:

- Break-up of some protein fibrillar matrix

- Opacities occurring in the degenerative vitreous of myopia

- Posterior vitreous detachment.

Break-up of the protein fibrillar matrix may produce typically fine opacities, but these may be so minute as to be barely visible or unseen with the ophthalmoscope. Traditionally, they are called 'flying flies', or muscae volitantes.

Opacities occurring in the degenerative vitreous of myopes are frequently noticed by the patient and are certainly easily seen by the examiner. It almost seems that the larger eye of the myope has more space within which the vitreous gel can disintegrate. Clouds of opacities may occur which can possibly obscure the vision temporarily.

Posterior vitreous detachment is a common clinical event in middle life, usually spontaneous but occasionally precipitated by trauma. The gel appears to collapse from behind so that an irregular ball of rather denser gel is gathered forward into the middle and anterior (retrolental) portion of the vitreous cavity. There is a distinct interface between the ball and the thinner, more fluid gel between the ball and the retina. This

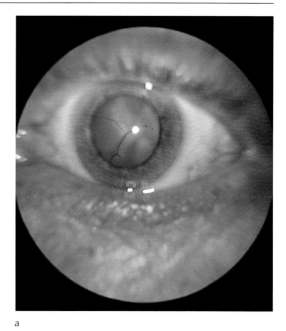

a

b

Figure 11.1 Two ophthalmoscopic views of a vitreous detachment, the eye having moved slightly between (*a*) and (*b*). Such opacities would have little effect on the visual acuity.

often contains an incomplete ring of opacity, which can be seen with the ophthalmoscope, where the interface has detached itself from its adhesion to the optic disc. The ring marks the site of the original attachment of the boundary of the vitreous body to the optic disc (Figure 11.1). The patient complains of the sudden appearance of one or more floating objects in the vision associated with flashes of light or sparks occurring very typically in the outer, temporal part of the field of vision.

In itself, posterior vitreous detachment is harmless but occasionally the interface membrane remains adherent to some pathological area of the retina which may lead to the formation of a hole and thence to a retinal detachment (see Chapter 12). It is unfortunately confusing, but true, that both spots and flashes of light may be symptomatic of the formation of a retinal hole. It is therefore important that the retina be fully examined in all patients presenting with these symptoms. Referral to an ophthalmologist is mandatory.

There is no treatment for posterior vitreous detachment, but if the retina is normal the patient can be reassured that the condition is not serious. The flashes of light usually disappear within three to four weeks, and though the opacity may continue to be visible for some time, it normally drops out of the line of vision and is mentally dismissed by the patient.

Inflammatory debris in the vitreous

The condition occurs as a result of posterior uveitis (see Chapter 9). An inflamed choroid may exude material through the retina into the vitreous. Such material may also arise from the posterior part (the pars plana) of the ciliary body in cyclitis. This produces floaters in the vision and the floaters may be so profuse and 'heavy' that the vision of the eye is seriously obscured.

Treatment is directed to the causal uveitis, but even when this has subsided — and because the vitreous has no throughflow — the opacities may still be present for several months before clearing.

Vitreous haemorrhage

This is an important condition. In its lesser form the patient complains merely of spots or floaters, or smoky vision. A much more severe version may cause sudden loss of sight (Figure 11.2).

The causes of vitreous haemorrhage fall roughly into two groups of pathology:

1 The vitreous haemorrhage arises from vascular pathology of the retina, either as a retinal haemorrhage itself or as some disorder of the retinal blood vessels (vascular retinopathy) such as that which occurs in diabetes (see page 223). Whether its origin be in exudative senile maculopathy, or trauma, or even that associated with subarachnoid haemorrhage, any retinal haemorrhage, if sufficiently large, may leak into the vitreous.

A rather uncommon disease of the peripheral retinal veins, periphlebitis, may give rise to recurrent vitreous haemorrhages, particularly in young men. It is known as Eales' disease.

2 The vitreous haemorrhage may occur in relation to the pathogenesis of retinal holes and detachments. The retina bleeds as the hole or a tear occurs.

A vitreous haemorrhage must therefore, in every instance, be considered from these two standpoints. Thus if the patient is diabetic, the first assumption must be that the haemorrhage results from diabetic retinopathy. However, in a patient who is a high myope and in good general health, a retinal tear with or without detachment must be suspected.

The diagnostic difficulty is aggravated by the fact that the haemorrhage may be so dense that the retina cannot be seen. It is therefore usual to wait and see if the haemorrhage absorbs itself. The patient should be advised to avoid physical exertion, even to take a few days' bedrest. If there is no sign of the haemorrhage clearing within two or three days, an ultrasound examination may be advisable to discover whether the retina has become detached.

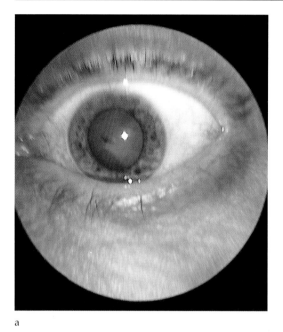

a

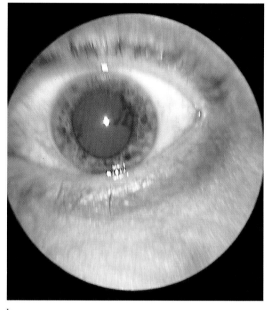

b

c

Figure 11.2   Three views of a vitreous haemorrhage, the eye having moved slightly between the views. A variable degree of obscuring of the vision occurs and would be particularly marked in (*c*).

The urgency here is to replace the detached retina. The surgical technique involves the ability to see where the retinal hole, or holes, actually are so they may be properly sealed (see page 105); but the blood in the vitreous makes this very difficult to do.

Prognosis and management   Most vitreous haemorrhages clear spontaneously, but often slowly, taking weeks or sometimes months.

In recent years it has become possible to evacuate a persisting vitreous haemorrhage by the special technique known as a vitrectomy. The vitreous is removed and replaced with saline or another fluid. The procedure is not usually undertaken early, unless there is an urgent reason to examine the fundus, for example if a retinal detachment is suspected.

All forms of vitreous haemorrhage, particularly those occurring in diabetics, may organize; that is to say, they may be replaced by fibrous tissue. The scar which forms attaches itself to the framework of the vitreous and to the retina (retinitis proliferans) and then shrinks and pulls away the retina, the so-called 'traction retinal detachment'. The condition is a less common variety of retinal detachment than the usual type referred to on page 102. It is more difficult to treat it surgically and its intractability can lead to the unfortunate end result found in some cases of diabetic retinopathy, with the sight being permanently lost.

PRACTICAL POINTS

● Differential diagnosis of change in the vitreous may be difficult and require specialist examination. Inflammatory debris and haemorrhages can be dense enough to obscure the red reflex obtained with the ophthalmoscope.

● Posterior vitreous detachment requires full examination of the retina to establish whether hole formation threatening retinal detachment has occurred.

● Vitreous haemorrhage may signify vascular disease affecting the retina or may arise from a retinal tear with the possible development of a retinal detachment. It may itself result in traction retinal detachment, a type which is especially difficult surgically.

12   Retinal disease

The retina lines the posterior two-thirds of the eyeball on which an inverted image of the outside world is formed. For example, the upper retina subserves the lower visual field and the nasal retina the temporal field of vision.

Light reaches the photosensitive elements, the rods and cones, by passing through its inner layers. At the posterior pole of the eye, the part of the retina responsible for central vision (the macula) shows modifications from the general microanatomy (Figures 12.1 and 12.2). At the macula, most of the inner layers are pushed aside to expose the sensitive cells more directly to light; these are mostly cones, which are responsible for day and colour vision. Elsewhere in the retina a mixture of cones and rods is found, the latter being responsible for night vision.

The photosensitive elements are on the outside surface of the retina, with their processes closely related to the pigment epithelium. The epithelium is separated from the capillary plexus of the choroid by a structureless lamina known as Bruch's membrane.

Both pigment epithelium and neural elements of the retina are developed from the primary optic vesicles, and are central nervous tissue in embryological origin. This is an important point in eye disease because any destruction of the retinal neurones is irreplaceable. In general, therefore, any visual loss due to such a pathology is likely to be permanent.

Another important fact about the retina is its dual nutrition. The inner layers of the retina have a true vascular supply: the central retinal artery, its branches and capillaries and collecting veins. The outer layers, which include rods and cones, are avascular and depend for their nutrition upon diffusion from the choroidal capillary circulation. The central artery is effectively an end artery and its occlusion leads to the death of the inner retinal layers.

Disturbance of the choroidal circulation is never more than patchy, as the blood supply of the choroid anastomoses with other vessels. However, the area of choroidal capillaries immediately under the macula is particularly prone to pathological events later in life (see page 98).

This chapter looks at two diseases of the outer retinal layers.

- Senile macular degeneration

- Retinal detachment.

The effects of vascular disease are discussed in Chapter 22.

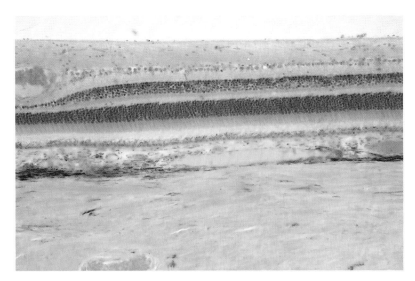

Figure 12.1 The general anatomy of the retina.

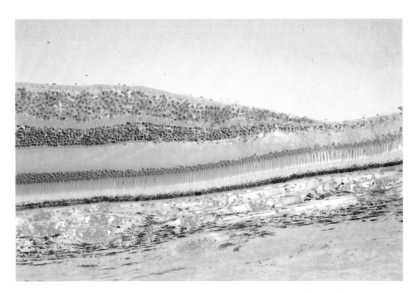

Figure 12.2 The specialized anatomy of the retina at one border of the macular area. The space separating the rods and cones from the dense pigmented epithelium is an artefact. Outside the pigment epithelium is the lightly pigmented choroid.

SENILE MACULAR DEGENERATION

As its name implies, senile macular degeneration is a degenerative condition of the macula occurring late in life; commonly over the age of sixty-five years. The vision of one or both eyes deteriorates, usually gradually, but, according to the type of degeneration (see below), the sight may occasionally be lost suddenly.

No treatment available is likely to improve the vision, although optical measures may help overcome the disability.

The rest of the retina is usually quite normal and though the patient will experience serious difficulty in reading and writing, the peripheral vision is retained. In fact, with care, the patient can move about independently, especially in familiar surroundings.

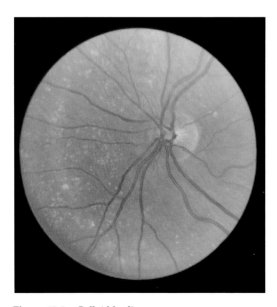

Figure 12.3   Colloid bodies.

The condition exists in two forms: exudative and dry. Bruch's membrane pathology is probably the basis of both forms, and may exist prior to visual deterioration. A common picture is of colloid bodies, or Drusen (Figure 12.3), which are yellowish-white punctate accumulations of what may be retinal debris in the membrane. The condition is usually symptomless. It is not necessarily a precursor of macular degeneration and may or may not be present in other parts of the retina. The colloid bodies are often misdiagnosed as exudates, but their appearance, and the absence of other signs such as those associated with vascular retinopathies (see page 219), serve to distinguish them.

Exudative forms of macular degeneration

In this form, leakage of fluid or blood between Bruch's membrane and the pigment epithelium will occur. This often arises from a neovascular membrane growing in from the choroidal circulation. The leakage may be acute, leading to a profound and sudden loss of vision, which happens because the central retina is disrupted; the macula appears grey and swollen with true exudate, or obvious haemorrhage, surrounding the elevation (Figures 12.4 and 12.5).

There is no treatment to help an established condition, and the central vision becomes permanently lost, although initially the complaint may simply be of distortion of objects. However, if the condition is diagnosed early, and particularly if the affected or the fellow eye shows an obvious subretinal vascular membrane, it may be possible to arrest or prevent loss of vision. To this end, two modern techniques are of some value. These are:

● Fluorescein retinal angiography

● Laser photocoagulation.

Fluorescein angiography   In this technique the dye, fluorescein, is injected intravenously into an

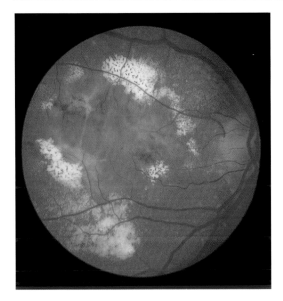

Figure 12.4   Exudative degeneration of the macula.

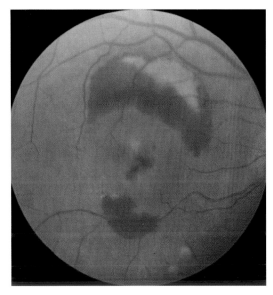

Figure 12.5   Macular haemorrhage.

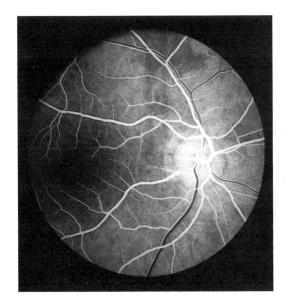

Figure 12.6   A normal fluorescein retinal angiogram. The fluorescing areas are white. In this picture all the arterioles are already filled and the veins are beginning to fill. The macular area is dark because in the normal retina no fluorescence appears.

arm vein. In the seconds that follow, photographs of the retina are taken at frequent intervals, every second or so (Figure 12.6). The system is so arranged that the illuminating light is of a wavelength that maximally excites fluorescence in the circulating dye and a filter allows into the camera only the wavelength of excited fluorescein.

In normal circumstances, an angiogram of the retina is obtained showing the fluorescence confined to the retinal blood vessels. In pathological conditions, the angiogram may show areas of closure of parts of the retinal capillary network. Such areas in the deep retinal network may be surrounded by microaneurysms: in the superficial layer, focal capillary closure may be found near cotton wool spots.

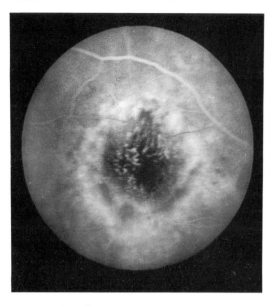

Figure 12.7   A fluorescein retinal angiogram in a case of senile exudative macular degeneration. There is a ring of fluorescence around a dark macular area. this central area contains exudate which masks deeper fluorescence.

If the endothelium of the normal or abnormal retinal vessels is incompetent, then leakage of fluorescein may occur. In the vascular retinopathies of hypertension and diabetes, this may be found in association with deep or superficial haemorrhage or near to hard (deep) exudates.

The leakage of fluorescein which occurs in senile macular degeneration, perhaps from an associated neovascular membrane (Figure 12.7), and in the condition of pigment epithelial detachment (see below), where safe to do so, may indicate a site suitable for laser treatment.

Laser treatment in senile macular degeneration
The elderly patient is usually unaware of the problem until the sight deteriorates, but if one eye has been affected, the patient will be alerted to the slightest deterioration or distortion of vision in the fellow eye. Prompt investigation and treatment by the laser (Figure 12.8) may help a minor proportion of cases of what is, in its more developed form, an untreatable condition.

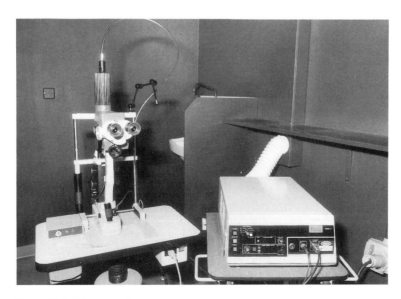

Figure 12.8   The argon laser.

It must be emphasized that the expectations of laser treatment in senile macular degeneration should not be pitched too high. In some cases the area requiring treatment may be so close to the foveal region of the macula that the burn produced by the laser will destroy what remains of the central vision. In other cases, the continuation of the pathological process, after laser therapy, sometimes leads patients to believe that the treatment actually encouraged deterioration.

A more extended account of the laser is given in the sections on retinal detachment and diabetic retinopathy, where this kind of treatment is of unquestioned and established value.

Dry forms of degeneration

In the dry form of macular degeneration, the pigment epithelium of the retina degenerates and there may be an associated localized sclerosis of the choroidal capillary plexus.

Some loss of central vision, which may be progressive, will occur (Figure 12.9). Irregular pigmentation, colloid bodies and tiny true exudates confined to the macular region are common features of the ophthalmic appearance.

Optical management in macular degeneration
Loss of vision due to macular causes may be improved by magnifying the retinal image so that the interpretable pieces fall on the normal retina surrounding the blind area. Simple magnifying glasses, telescopic spectacles and projection devices such as closed-circuit television, are all helpful. However, success depends on the patient's motivation to persist in trying to overcome an inevitable disability, as well as on the degree of degeneration that has occurred.

It is most important to reassure patients that however bad they believe their vision to be, they will never go blind. These patients should be encouraged to do any reading they can manage, with the print held very close, and be assured that this is not harmful. Similarly, these patients may sit as close as possible to their television screens, if this gives them a better picture.

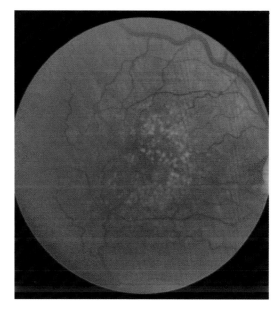

Figure 12.9   The dry form of senile macular degeneration.

Other forms of macular pathology

Apart from the usual macular changes in old age, the macula may be selectively involved in other conditions, particularly high myopia. Two other conditions should be noted:

● At all ages a detachment of the pigment epithelium may occur in the macular region of otherwise normal subjects, producing a sudden deterioration of the sight (Figure 12.10). Some degree of spontaneous improvement may be possible if the fluid accumulation associated with this is slight, and no severe destruction of the cones has occurred.

● Even without pigment epithelium pathology, a curious condition of selective oedema of the macula occurs, usually in young adults,

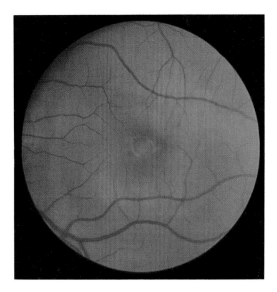

Figure 12.10   Pigment epithelial detachment.

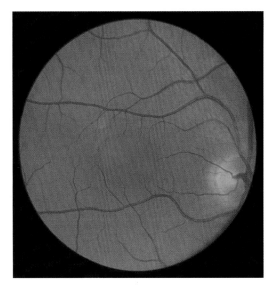

Figure 12.11   Central serous retinopathy.

known as central serous retinopathy (Figure 12.11). Typically the patient complains of a grey disc of discoloration over whatever is looked at directly by the affected eye. The ophthalmoscope shows a grey macula surrounded by a circular ring of reflected light. The usual course of this condition is that it resolves itself over a period of weeks or months. Fluorescein retinal angiography may show no abnormality, but occasionally reveals an area of fluorescein leakage, the sealing of which by photocoagulation may help abbreviate the course of the condition. Its cause is unknown.

RETINAL DETACHMENT

Retinal detachment is the collective term for conditions in which there is displacement of the retina from its normal position. There is only one common variety, a simple retinal detachment.

Primary simple retinal detachment

Primary retinal displacement occurs when fluid accumulates between the pigment epithelium and the remainder of the retina (incidentally re-establishing the cavity of the primary optic vesicle). This separates the rods and cones from contact with their source of nutrition, leaving them functionless even if they do not die.

Symptoms and signs of retinal detachment   It follows that the parts of the retina that are detached are blind, the main symptom being a field defect usually described as a shadow corresponding to the detached area. The natural history of a retinal detachment is for the detachment to extend so that the shadow becomes gradually larger. Eventually the macula is stripped off, the shadow engulfing the central vision, which is then lost.

The detached retina, as viewed through the ophthalmoscope, has the following characteristics (Figure 12.12):

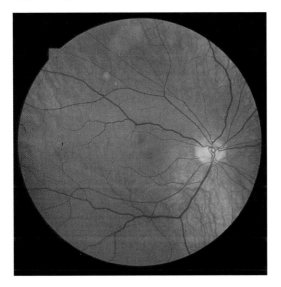

Figure 12.12 Retinal detachment; the lower left retina is grey and the vessels on its surface wrinkled.

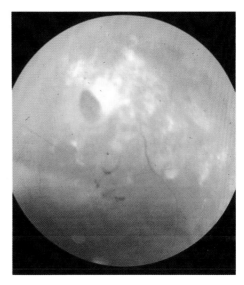

Figure 12.13 A retinal hole.

● A grey and wrinkled appearance which may undulate as the eye moves

● The vessels appear dark, narrow and tortuous; this is because they are no longer in close contact with the red glow given by the choroidal vascular background, which is responsible for the normal red reflex seen with the ophthalmoscope.

● One or more retinal holes may be visible in the detached area of the retina (Figure 12.13).

Binocular indirect ophthalmoscopy This is a routine but specialized method of retinal inspection of particular value in detachment work (Figure 12.14). A stereoscopic and brightly lit inverted image of the retina is inspected with both eyes; the field of view is larger than that obtained by conventional direct ophthalmoscopy, the image being correspondingly smaller.

The stereoscopic element is particularly helpful in identifying levels in the view obtained, making it easier to assess the extent of detachment of the retina.

The mechanism of simple retinal detachment
The fluid of a simple retinal detachment achieves its subretinal position by passing from the vitreous through holes or tears in the retina. These occur in the following patients:

1 High myopes with large eyes and stretched retinae. There may be a family history not

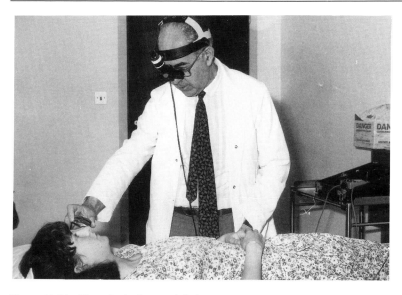

Figure 12.14   Binocular indirect ophthalmoscopy.

only of myopia, but also of retinal detachment itself.

2 Elderly patients with degeneration in the periphery of the retina.

3 Traumatized patients: this group includes those patients who have had severe blunt injuries or penetrating injuries with loss of vitreous, as well as cataract surgery patients.

The development of a hole or tear is an independent event and is not necessarily followed by fluid passing through the hole to cause a detachment, even though this is the usual sequel.

The process of hole formation may be symptomless, but the patient sometimes experiences flashes of light and perhaps spots in the vision. The spots may be a sign of vitreous haemorrhage coming from the torn retina. It is important to remember that these spots may also be a symptom of a vitreous detachment (see Chapter 11) which is usually an innocent condition, but may occasionally itself be the initiating cause of a retinal tear.

Management of retinal detachment Retinal detachment is best treated as an emergency because of the imminent possibility of the detachment extending to involve the macula, if it has not already done so at presentation. Detachment of the macula always worsens the prognosis for recovery of vision, even after successful surgery; upper retinal detachment is especially likely to detach the macula because of the downward gravitation of the subretinal fluid. Any patient in whom this is recognized should be laid down flat prior to and during transportation to the hospital.

Almost without exception, the treatment of retinal detachment is surgical. In some cases, preoperative bedrest may assist the fluid to re-enter the vitreous cavity, from where it came, via the hole. The retina occasionally flattens comple-tely, but without some operative intervention it simply detaches itself again, once the patient becomes mobilized.

A full examination of the retina of both eyes is important because, if there are any holes present without retinal detachment, prophylactic surgery may be necessary for the unaffected eye.

Surgical treatment of retinal detachment is directed primarily to the localization and closure of retinal holes or tears with, in some cases, evacuation of the subretinal fluid.

Closure of retinal holes In established retinal detachment this is effected by bringing the area of the retina in which the holes are present into contact with part of the choroid that has been made 'tacky' by inflammation. In most cases, the inflammation is produced by cryotherapy, cer-tainly if an established detachment is present (Figure 12.15). The classical but now outmoded method of making the choroid inflamed was to apply heat, usually diathermy, to the appropri-ate area.

Restoration of the retina to its position in contact with the choroid In order to ensure that the detached retina settles on to the prepared choroid, it is customary to indent the sclera by suturing silicone 'explants' to it (Figure 12.16), or encircling the globe with a silicone band. This produces obvious internal bulges carrying the choroid towards the retina. By strategic place-ment of these bulges the retinal hole or holes will

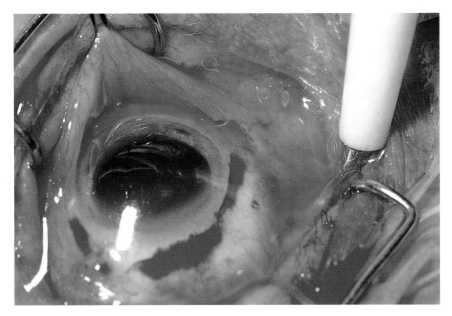

Figure 12.15 Cryotherapy being applied to the retina through the sclera while the retina is inspected with the binocular ophthalmoscope.

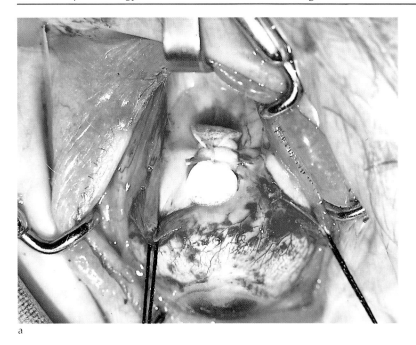

a

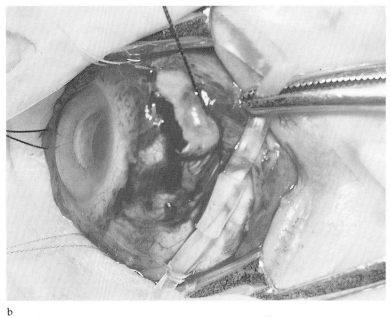

b

Figure 12.16   Two types of explant: (*a*) a silicone
plomb has been stitched to the sclera; (*b*) the ends of
an encircling band are being joined together. The band
extends right around the globe.

be brought into contact with the 'sticky' choroid even if some fluid separating retina and choroid remains elsewhere. If the holes are sealed, this fluid beneath the retina will often absorb spontaneously. In other cases, the fluid needs to be evacuated to allow the hole to seal and the retina to return to its normal position.

Air, special gas, or silicone oil may be introduced into the vitreous to push the retina on to the choroid. In certain complex cases, total removal of the vitreous may be necessary so as to attack any abnormal adhesions of the internal retina that would prevent its returning to a normal position. In these procedures, the sealing of the retinal hole is normally carried out with the laser.

Closure of retinal holes by laser and photocoagulation If a retinal hole is present without detachment, phototherapy either by laser or xenon arc photocoagulator may be sufficient to provide the localized inflammation of the choroid. The principle of the treatment is as follows. The pigment in the outer epithelium of the retina normally absorbs light that is passed through the transparent neural layers. Indeed, one of its functions is to act as a 'back' to the photographic plate to prevent a diffusion of the image which might otherwise occur. This does happen in congenital defects of pigmentation such as albinism, where defective vision is associated with nystagmus and with 'pink' irides as the fundus red reflex comes back through the iris.

If powerful light reaches the pigment epithelium, it will lead to the generation of excessive amounts of heat and a localized burn will occur. The clinical condition of eclipse blindness is an example of this. Here the full force of solar energy lands on the macula as the sun emerges from behind the moon. It is for this reason that direct viewing of an eclipse, with whatever 'protection', is inadvisable.

The burn is, however, made use of clinically in many ophthalmic conditions. Its original use was in the treatment of retinal detachment where, as mentioned above, the principle of management is to close retinal holes by production of inflammation in the choroid, which then seals the overlying retina. If holes are present that are not yet associated with detachment, the retina is still in contact with the choroid and an intense light from either a laser or xenon arc photocoagulator can produce the appropriate local burn without recourse to an invasive technique. The xenon arc coagulator is simply a very powerful light source. The laser derives its extraordinary power from the coherence of its radiation.

Other types of retinal detachment

Generally, other types of retinal detachment are uncommon, but two deserve special mention:

● Traction detachment, associated with organized vitreous haemorrhage, is a particular feature of advanced diabetic retinopathy. Its successful management is difficult and, from a visual standpoint, often unrewarding.

● The retina may be displaced by a tumour of the choroid. A malignant melanoma is the usual cause, but secondary deposits from breast carcinoma are occasionally responsible. Some of the distinguishing features are shown in Figure 12.17a. The differential diagnosis is important, and the absence of a retinal hole together with the solid (as distinct from fluid) appearance of at least part of the detachment are significant findings.

At one time it was advised that an eye with a suspected malignant melanoma (which may also occur in the ciliary body or the iris) be removed. This may still be true for large tumours occupying, say, a quarter of the globe, particularly if the central vision is affected (Figure 12.17b). Now, however, with smaller neoplasms, the view is that surgical removal may encourage metastasis, so a 'watching brief' policy is usually adopted.

Radiotherapy has some part to play in attempting to eradicate tumours of this nature, especially when it does not affect the macula and the central vision remains good. The technique,

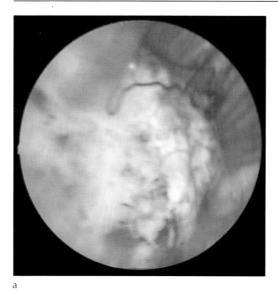

a

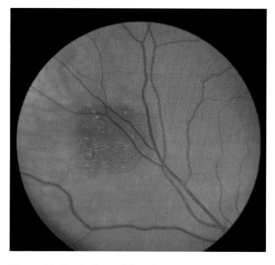

Figure 12.18   A choroidal mole.

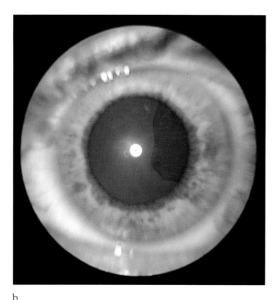

b

Figure 12.17   Malignant melanomas of the choroid: (*a*) the appearance is that of a retinal detachment; (*b*) a large black shadow, indicating a tumour occupying perhaps a quarter of the globe, interferes with the red reflex.

although particularly applicable to the retinal tumour (often familial) of infancy and childhood, the retinoblastoma, is now sometimes used even for malignant melanomas of the choroid. Secondary deposits in the choroid, arising most commonly from the dissemination of breast cancer, respond well to external irradiation.

As with malignant melanomas occurring elsewhere in the body, those in the choroid continue to have a reputation for early metastasis. Cases similar to that of the classical 'glass eye plus large liver' are still encountered today.

Benign choroidal melanoma is however a very much more common condition (Figure 12.18). It rarely goes on to malignancy.

Other retinal degenerations

Retinitis pigmentosa

This classical condition is not uncommon. It is basically an inherited disorder of the sensory elements of the retina, possibly related to a genetic biochemical abnormality. The inheritance is of diverse forms, but the sex-linked recessive mode is common.

The rods are first affected, the cones later on, so poor night vision is a common presentation. The paucity of rods at the macula means that the central vision is spared until late in the disease, but early on a profound loss of visual field occurs. The visual field eventually shrinks so much that what remains allows only tunnel vision (see Chapter 24).

Diagnosis is usually made from the history of night blindness and the typical retinal appearance, as well as by a characteristic restriction of the visual field:

1 The retina shows 'bone corpuscle' shaped clumps of pigment in the non-central areas, starting in the mid-periphery and giving rise to the characteristic ring scotoma in the visual field found in the early stage. The pigment is released following secondary degeneration of the retinal pigment epithelium (Figure 12.19).

2 The arteries are often attenuated with waxy, pale optic discs.

3 Cataract may develop later in life and successful surgery for this may restore central vision, even in advanced cases with a very reduced visual field.

4 Total blindness is uncommon, but is found more often in cases where the clinical onset was early in life.

5 Early recognition of the condition is possibly from the electroretinogram (ERG). This is a small potential (about 0.5 mV) which is generated between the cornea and an indifferent electrode if the retina is exposed to a flash of light. A biphasic or monophasic response is obtained according to whether or not the light is bright or dim. The ERG is likely to indicate gross retinal dysfunction if it is disturbed or absent and in conditions such as retinitis pigmentosa or in certain other congenital degenerations of the retina, the absence of the ERG may be one of the earliest signs of the condition, even before ophthalmoscopic signs appear.

Patients diagnosed early in life need advice on the type of occupation or career they should aim for, the specialist organizations that may help, and the local authority arrangements available to them. It is sensible for a parent, or potential parent with the condition (as well as parents of children who are known sufferers) to be referred for genetic counselling.

Treatment is ineffective. Whatever claims are made for such measures as pituitary extract ('intermedin' is a pigment controller), placental extract, or vasodilators, they usually turn out to be spurious: the natural course of the disease often includes long periods of stability before further deterioration occurs.

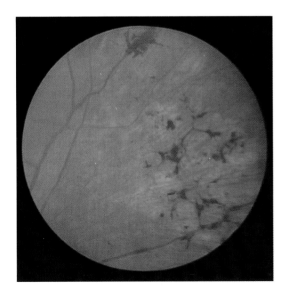

Figure 12.19 Retinitis pigmentosa.

PRACTICAL POINTS

● Senile macular degeneration is one of the three common causes of failing vision in old age. It presents as a dry or as an exudative form.

● Treatment is usually ineffective, but in a very small proportion of cases of exudative senile macular degeneration diagnosed early enough, progression may be successfully arrested by laser treatment.

● Visual aids include a magnifying glass, but any form of aid is only as effective as the patient's motivation in using it. The practitioner should give all encouragement possible.

● Simple retinal detachment is the only common form, characteristically occurring in high myopes, elderly or traumatized patients. The symptom is a defect of the visual field appearing as a shadow, progressing to loss of the central sight.

● Retinal detachment should be treated as an emergency, almost invariably requiring surgery.

● An uncommon but important type of detachment of the retina is that produced by malignancies of the choroid, a primary melanoma or a secondary deposit frequently from a breast primary.

● There is no treatment for retinitis pigmentosa. Patients may need advice on adjusting their lifestyles to the condition.

● Genetic counselling should be given in appropriate cases.

13 Glaucomas

Glaucomas (note the plural) is the term used to describe many conditions in which high eye pressure produces undesirable effects on the eye and sight. Glaucoma is not a single disease.

When a patient is diagnosed as having 'glaucoma', it usually means that he has one of two particular conditions, the primary glaucomas, which are:

- Chronic simple glaucoma, open angle glaucoma being the alternative name
- Closed angle glaucoma.

Chronic simple glaucoma is much commoner than the closed angle variety. The other glaucomas are the secondary types in which the rise in eye pressure is due to some other eye condition. These types of glaucoma are not described in great detail here, although the important ones are mentioned elsewhere as complications of these conditions (see Chapters 9, 10 and 22).

Intraocular pressure

Measurement of the intraocular pressure

Simple palpation (Figure 13.1) can give a crude and clinical estimate of the hardness of the eye. This is not a particularly reliable method, but is useful for comparing the pressure of the two eyes. Of the various instrumental methods of measuring the pressure, most give approximately similar absolute readings in millimetres of mercury. Applanation tonometry is the most reliable method (Figure 13.2). Non-contact tonometry, using a 'puff of air' on to the cornea is less accurate.

Normal and abnormal intraocular pressure

The normal intraocular pressure is a resultant of the inflow and outflow of aqueous humour. The aqueous is produced by the ciliary processes and passes between the front of the lens and the iris, then through the pupil into the anterior chamber (Figure 13.3). From the anterior chamber, it passes out of the eye via the 'anterior chamber angle', which is formed by the root of the iris and the cornea, and then percolates through to the canal of Schlemm. This circular channel is situated at the edge of the cornea; its inner wall through which the aqueous passes, consists of a pore-like meshwork called the 'trabeculum' or the 'trabecular tissue'. The aqueous leaves the canal of Schlemm by special vessels and joins the venous circulation, thus entering the blood from which it originated.

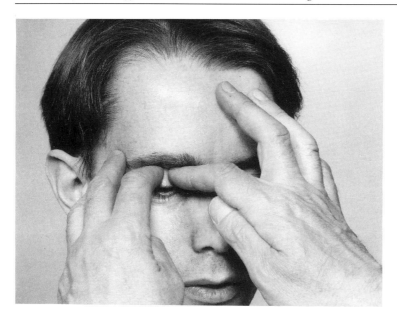

Figure 13.1   Digital tonometry.

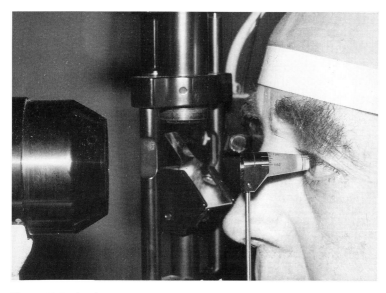

Figure 13.2   Applanation tonometry.

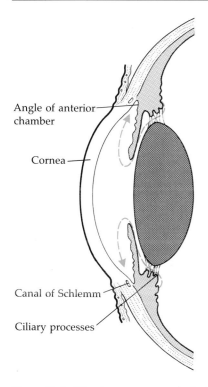

Angle of anterior chamber

Cornea

Canal of Schlemm

Ciliary processes

Figure 13.3 The structures concerned with the formation, circulation and drainage of aqueous humour.

The balance between the input and outflow of aqueous humour maintains a pressure within the eyeball, which is sufficient to keep it a regular and fixed shape, so allowing it to function as a precise optical instrument. The aqueous humour also has a nutritional function for the avascular structures it comes in contact with, for example, the lens and the cornea.

The balance of inflow and outflow of aqueous humour is not so precise as to be able to say that any particular eye pressure is normal. Measurement of the eye pressure on a series of patients will give a variable range, but the indication is that in middle life a pressure of 20 mmHg or less

may be accepted as being normal. It is unusual to find people with extremely low eye pressure. Statistically the average is approximately 16.5 mmHg.

In most cases of glaucoma, the intraocular pressure is indisputably higher than 20 mmHg in the untreated eye.

CHRONIC SIMPLE GLAUCOMA: OPEN ANGLE GLAUCOMA

To the non-specialist the term glaucoma has dramatic associations. Unfortunately, however, chronic simple glaucoma has very little drama about it until it is quite advanced, when loss of sight occurs in a painless and uninflamed eye.

What appears to happen is that over a period of years the ocular pressure rises steadily. The precise cause is unknown, but it is generally agreed that the problem is one of an obstructed outflow of aqueous humour, rather than excessive production. The exact site of the obstruction is unclear. Some believe it is in the trabeculum, its pore-like spaces being reduced. Others consider that the connections between the canal of Schlemm and the venous circulation are in some way sclerosed.

At a certain level, which is by no means absolute and which varies from patient to patient, the optic disc begins to alter, indicating malfunction or death of some of the constituent nerve fibres. Ophthalmoscopically the alteration can be seen as a 'cupping' of the disc. The appearance is as if the disc, which is of course the optic nerve head, is being expelled from the eye by the heightened pressure (see Figures 13.4–13.7). Untreated, the pressure may cause total atrophy of the optic nerve and result in irreversible blindness.

Symptoms

The symptoms of chronic simple glaucoma relate solely to those fibres of the optic nerve which become functionless due to the glaucomatous process. If the fibres come from a part of the

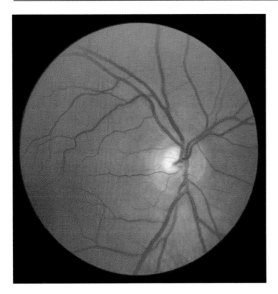

Figure 13.4 Physiological cupping of the disc.

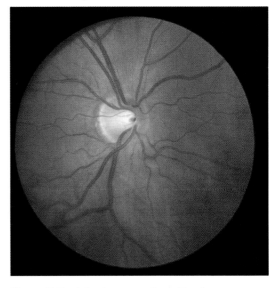

Figure 13.5 A further example, with a larger cup.

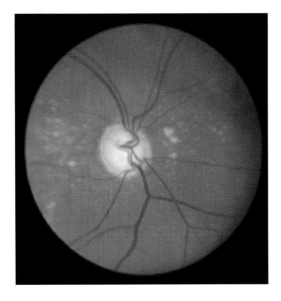

Figure 13.6 A glaucomatous cupped disc.

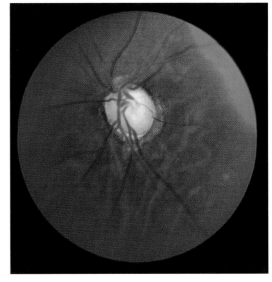

Figure 13.7 A very advanced glaucomatous cupped disc. Note the extreme pallor.

retina responsible for a peripheral portion of the visual field, the patient may be unaware of any functional defect. This is especially so if, as commonly occurs, loss of the nasal visual field is an early event and the patient's fellow eye is unaffected or less advanced. Loss of temporal field is noticed much earlier and it is only when the loss of function extends to the central retinal fibres, the papillomacular bundle, that a defect becomes noticeable in the central vision. In other words, the commonest symptom of chronic simple glaucoma is failing sight.

Diagnosis

Diagnosis of chronic simple glaucoma may be made during an eye examination for symptoms such as those just described above. However, the condition may be found in a routine inspection of the fundus, as part of a general medical or ophthalmological examination. Cupping of the optic disc, for example, is the important sign. The appearance of the optic disc may be convincingly glaucomatous or be simply a varient of normal physiological cupping. In all such cases, charting of the visual field is essential.

Another route by which chronic simple glaucoma may be discovered is through routine tonometry, and this brings us to the subject of prevention.

Early recognition and prevention

The tragedy of unrecognized chronic simple glaucoma, and therefore the chances of prevention or amelioration, are now better understood. If the process is recognized before the optic atrophy has occurred, or has significantly progressed, treatment can arrest any further deterioration and the effects of chronic simple glaucoma thus be mitigated. The clinical problem would seem to be easily solved if every patient's intraocular pressure were measured in middle life (at which time chronic simple glaucoma becomes most common), as is done for blood

pressure. (It should be noted that intraocular pressure and blood pressure are not related.)

There is considerable difficulty in interpreting the results of mass population surveys of intraocular pressure, if 20 mmHg is taken to be the upper limit of normal pressure; what of the patient with a pressure of 25 mmHg whose optic disc is normal, as are his vision and visual field? Is it likely that this patient will develop chronic simple glaucoma, or is this 'highish' pressure simply a normal variant? The answer is not known and so the recommended course of action is observation, probably without treatment.

A mass survey could of course find actual cases of chronic simple glaucoma with established raised intraocular pressure, cupping of the optic disc and field loss. However, it is nonsense to label and treat as a case of chronic simple glaucoma a patient whose sole anomaly is that his intraocular pressure is slightly above the accepted norm.

Are surveys worthwhile? It is certainly important that the relatives of patients with known chronic simple glaucoma have regular ophthalmological examination in their middle years, as they are particularly likely to develop the condition.

Whether it is worthwhile for everyone to have a routine tonometry performed at the age of forty-five years, and at regular intervals thereafter, has not been conclusively established. The ideal is for the facility to be offered in conjunction with a sight test but it is at least as important for patients to be aware of the limitations of sight testing, and to regard as very serious any defects of their vision which the wearing of spectacles does not correct. It is equally important for every inspector of the fundus, ophthalmologist, optician, general practitioner or some other specialist, to be suspicious of optic disc appearances suggesting abnormal cupping.

Assessment

The patient with chronic simple glaucoma has virtually no symptoms other than a defect in

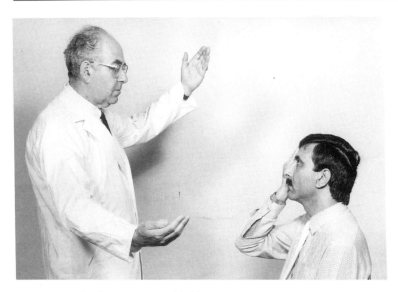

Figure 13.8   Confrontation visual fields.

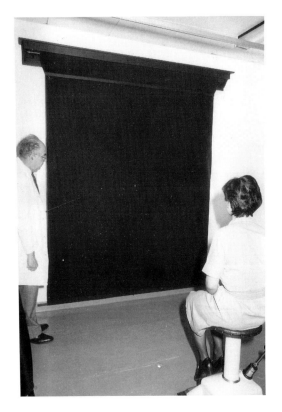

vision, unless the field of vision is very restricted. To the ophthalmologist, however, while central vision is a prime consideration, assessment also includes measurement of the intraocular pressure and estimation of the visual field, both of which need constant re-evaluation during the patient's follow-up.

The intraocular pressure may need repeated measurement because it often rises at different times of the day. For example, in the afternoon the patient may have a pressure of, say, below 20 mmHg, but in the early morning the measurement may be much higher.

Figure 13.9   The Bjerrum screen. The patient sits 2 m away and, using one eye at a time, fixes on the central white dot while the observer moves in hand-held white objects until the patient is able to see them.

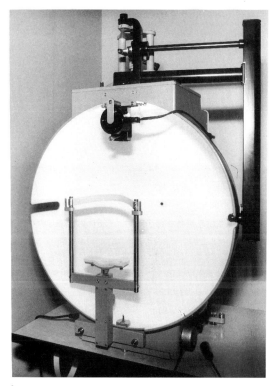

Figure 13.10   (*a*) The Goldmann perimeter and (*b*) the Friedmann visual field analyser. These are the instruments for the two standard types of perimetry, or visual field assessment. The Goldmann is a dynamic perimeter, the patient fixing on the centre of the bowl and the examiner moving an object towards the centre. The place where the object is first seen is recorded. The Friedmann analyser uses fixed points in the field, which are serially illuminated; the patient indicates whether or not he can see the spots of light. This is static perimetry.

The method of assessing the visual field varies from simple confrontation, which is actually valueless unless the field of loss is gross, to quite complex methods which allow automatic recordings of the limits of the field of vision (Figures 13.8–13.13).

Gonioscopy shows that the angle of the anterior chamber is unobstructed, hence the alternative name 'open angle' glaucoma (Figure 13.14).

a

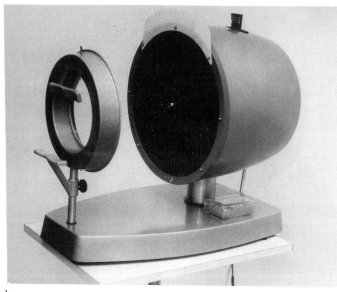

b

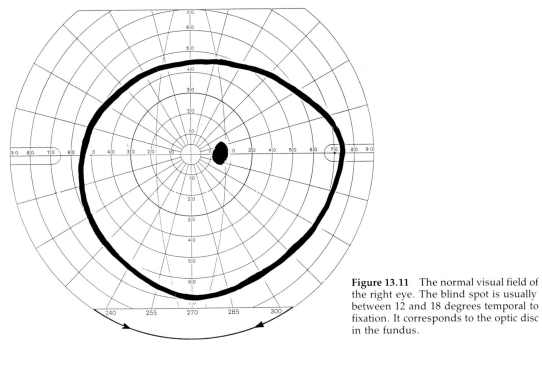

Figure 13.11 The normal visual field of the right eye. The blind spot is usually between 12 and 18 degrees temporal to fixation. It corresponds to the optic disc in the fundus.

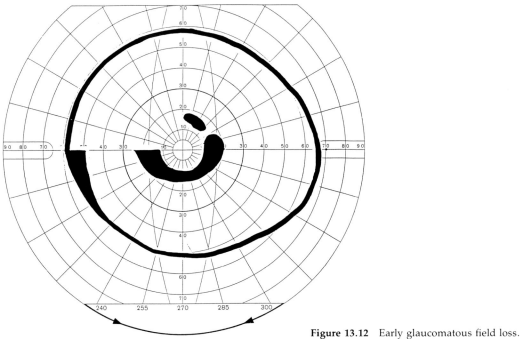

Figure 13.12 Early glaucomatous field loss.

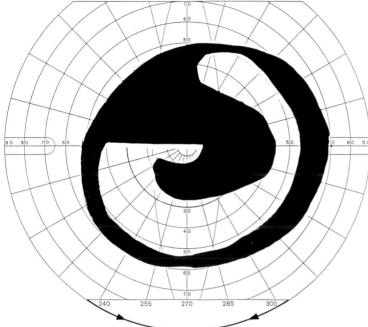

Figure 13.13   More advanced glaucomatous field loss.

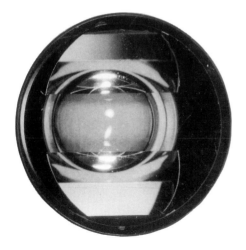

Figure 13.14   The gonioscope. This is a contact lens with incorporated mirror, which throws light into and allows observation at the angle of the anterior chamber.

Medical treatment

Eye drops (Table 13.1)   As mentioned, it is not known why the intraocular pressure rises in chronic simple glaucoma, though it is generally accepted that the abnormality is a restriction of the outflow of aqueous humour from the eye. Treatment is usually directed at improving the outflow; parasympathomimetic drugs, given as eyedrops, are believed to make this easier. This is the main medical treatment for the condition; commonly pilocarpine drops in strengths from 0.5 to 4 per cent (sometimes more) are given four times daily. Less well tolerated drugs are physostigmine, neostigmine, carbachol and phospholine iodide. All these drugs constrict the pupil and are known as the miotics. It should be noted that the miosis is only an indication that the drug has entered the eye, and does not signify that the patient's eye pressure is normal.

Table 13.1 Drops for chronic simple glaucoma.

Pharmacological group	Typical drop	Strength	Frequency
Parasympathomimetic	pilocarpine	0.5 to 4%	Four times daily
Sympathomimetic	adrenaline	0.5 or 1%	Twice daily
Ganglion blocker	guanethidine	1 to 5%	Twice daily
Beta-blocker	timolol	0.25 or 0.5%	Twice daily

It is uncertain how the drugs work against the condition. Possible modes of action are (1) by some direct effect in widening the 'pores' of the trabecular tissue (2) by stimulation of the ciliary muscle or (3) by a vascular effect on the outflow channels from the canal of Schlemm or on the plexus of blood vessels with which these channels connect.

Other eyedrops include adrenaline (0.5 or 1 per cent used twice daily), which may reduce the production of aqueous humour, ganglion blockers (guanethidine, 3 or 5 per cent) used twice daily, or beta-blockers of which the best known is timolol, 0.25 or 0.5 per cent, used twice daily; others include carteolol (1 and 2 per cent) and betaxolol (0.5 per cent).

The action of the beta-blockers in glaucoma is obscure, but it is believed that they also act on the input side, that is, they reduce the production of aqueous humour. They may all be used alone or in combination with other drops.

No matter which eyedrops are given, they must be used on a continual basis. Patients must be advised not to allow their supply to run out. Eye pressure will return to untreated levels within hours of discontinuing the drops.

Side-effects of eyedrops used for glaucoma
Pilocarpine has few side-effects and can be taken for years. Stronger parasympathomimetic drugs may not be so well tolerated. This group of drugs may be unsuitable for younger patients in whom accommodation is still active because the drugs send the ciliary muscle into contraction, thus producing an artificial myopia and some aching pain. The small pupil produced by the drugs sometimes gives rise to the complaint of diminishing or darkening of the vision.

In the younger age groups, slow release preparations of pilocarpine may be used, the ciliary spasm being less violent. These pellicles are placed in the upper conjunctival fornix and renewed weekly (Ocuserts).

Patients using adrenaline and guanethidine often develop very red eyes, which may lead to discomfort and are certainly unsightly. Because of this, some patients may be deterred from continuing to use these drugs. A pro-drug of adrenaline, dipivefrine (0.1 per cent), is thought to be equally effective with less unpleasant side-effects.

The continued use of drops containing adrenaline may lead to the deposition of pigment clumps on the conjunctival lining of the eyelids, especially the lower lid.

Timolol eyedrops may cause some loss of corneal sensitivity. They may also be systemically absorbed and slow the pulse. They are contraindicated in patients with bronchial asthma.

Acetazolamide   The long-term use of acetazolamide, a diuretic, in doses of 250 mg to 1000 mg daily, given orally, is a helpful added therapy. The drug is a carbonic anhydrase inhibitor, the enzyme being needed for the production of aqueous humour. Patients often complain of a tingling in the fingers or indigestion apart from the diuresis. Prolonged use of the drug may occasionally lead to a lowering of serum potassium; for this reason potassium supplements are sometimes given routinely for patients on long-term acetazolamide.

Surgery

Drainage procedures (Figure 13.15) are indicated where progression of chronic simple glaucoma is diagnosed on follow-up, particularly if the patient's intraocular pressure is uncontrolled and there is deteriorating visual function in either field of vision, or visual acuity.

If surgery is successful, the intraocular pressure will be reduced to a normal level. Postoperative inflammation may temporarily require mydriatics and steroid drops. The degree of pressure-lowering brought about by surgery is sometimes insufficient and so the medical therapy outlined above may have to be resumed. If this proves inadequate, further surgery may need to be considered.

Laser treatment   Marginally uncontrolled pressure may be reduced with laser treatment to the inner wall of the canal of Schlemm, and is often undertaken as a primary procedure. How this

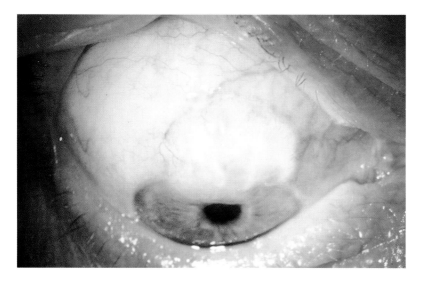

Figure 13.15   A glaucoma drainage operation; the patient is looking down and a bleb is present at the top margin of the cornea. This is the conjunctiva raised up by the aqueous humour draining through an artificially created fistula from the anterior chamber. The aqueous is absorbed into the conjunctival blood vessels of the bleb.

technique works is not known. If the intraocular pressure is not lowered to normal, the laser treatment may reduce it to a point where medical therapy may be more effective.

Prognosis of chronic simple glaucoma

In chronic simple glaucoma the loss of the visual field, if it has occurred at all, is permanent. Further loss can be prevented in moderate or early cases by keeping the pressure at a normal level with drops or other medication, or by surgery or laser therapy, or a combination of all three.

In advanced cases, where the field loss is very extensive when first diagnosed, the prognosis is poor with any form of treatment. The progression to blindness – absolute glaucoma – is often inevitable. Hence the strong argument for early diagnosis of the condition by routine measurement of the eye pressure during middle age or, even better, by informed inspection of the optic disc. (The term absolute glaucoma is widely used to refer to total loss of vision owing to any form of glaucoma, primary or secondary.)

Steroid eyedrops and glaucoma

The prolonged use of steroid eyedrops in certain susceptible individuals may cause a rise in ocular pressure and may eventually lead to a condition indistinguishable from chronic simple glaucoma. It is therefore important that special care is taken to avoid indiscriminate use of steroid eyedrops for patients with chronic red eyes of an indeterminate cause, or allergic conditions. Relatives of patients who have established chronic simple glaucoma are especially prone to develop a rise in ocular pressure in response to local steroid drops.

Atropine and chronic simple glaucoma

Chronic simple glaucoma is not affected by the administration of atropine. The obstruction to

the outflow of aqueous humour in the condition is not caused by the iris blocking the access of the aqueous humour to the canal of Schlemm; the angle of the anterior chamber is usually wide open so that dilatation of the pupil, by whatever means, is irrelevant to the condition.

Systemically administered drugs given for general disease often have an atropine-like action, and it is for this reason that they are marked 'contraindicated in glaucoma'. They can be given with impunity in chronic simple glaucoma, but should not be used in patients with the other type of primary glaucoma, the closed angle variety of glaucoma, which we consider next.

CLOSED ANGLE GLAUCOMA

This dramatic form of glaucoma is one which the medical student is always in fear of inducing or failing to recognize. In its acute form, closed angle glaucoma is part of the differential diagnosis of the acute red eye (see Chapter 3). In its intermittent or subacute form, the condition may present considerable diagnostic problems. It is also known as narrow angle glaucoma.

Anatomical basis

The anatomical basis for closed angle glaucoma is a certain shape of the anterior segment of the eye. In the susceptible eye, the angle of the anterior chamber is narrow, the iris being close to the cornea (see Figure 13.16). Such eyes may be small in their overall dimensions and are often hypermetropic. Even to the non-specialist, the anterior chamber may be seen to be shallow (Figure 13.17). In this setting the dilatation of the pupil is accompanied by a thickening of the peripheral part of the iris, which contacts the back edge of the cornea and blocks the access of the aqueous humour to the canal of Schlemm. The angle of the anterior chamber is therefore closed, hence the name of the condition. A patient with this susceptibility is likely to have a

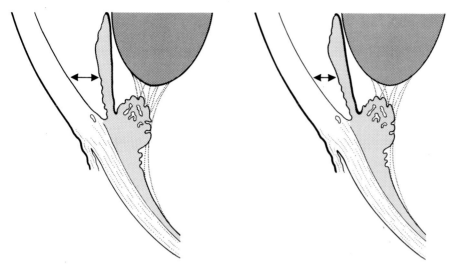

Figure 13.16   Cross sections of narrow and normal width anterior chamber angles (see also Figure 13.17).

shallow anterior chamber of both eyes so that bilateral acute glaucoma is always a possibility.

The relationship to pupillary dilatation explains the intermittent nature of the subacute form of the condition. The circumstances which produce these subacute attacks are precisely those which induce pupillary dilatation:

1 Darkness, or at least reduced illumination

2 Emotion

3 Drugs, particularly of the atropine-like variety administered to the eye for diagnostic or therapeutic purposes; very occasionally systemic administration has a similar effect.

Symptoms

In a dim or dark environment, an anatomically predisposed patient will experience pain, misty vision and haloes, coloured rings or rainbows around lights, particularly white car headlights. These are all symptoms of a sudden rise in intraocular pressure. The pain is in the eye, brow or temple. Oedema of the cornea occurs, leading to misty vision and haloes, the latter being the effect of epithelial droplets breaking up white light into its spectral components.

Many such attacks resolve spontaneously after a few hours (the pupil becoming smaller and the angle opening) and are often incorrectly attributed to migraine, especially as the pain from the eye may be regarded as a unilateral headache. It should be remembered that the visual phenomena of migraine are unrelated to external stimulation and that glaucomatous haloes are seen only around actual light.

Subacute closed angle glaucoma   Such attacks, known as subacute closed angle glaucoma, may

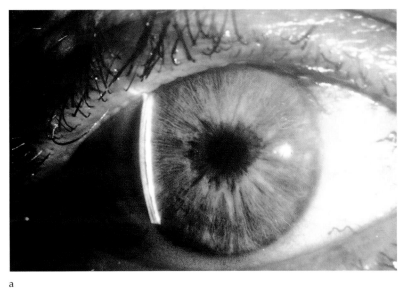

a

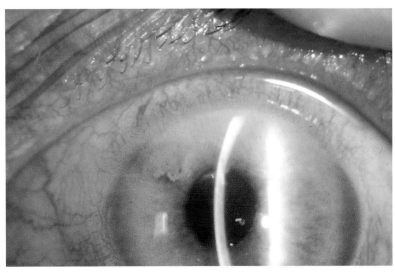

b

Figure 13.17   Slit-lamp appearances of (*a*) shallow and
(*b*) deep anterior chambers.

occur repeatedly. The effect of these rises of pressure on the optic nerve is not necessarily serious and attacks resolve spontaneously when the patient's pupil becomes small. However, most patients who experience repeated attacks of subacute glaucoma eventually end up with acute closed angle glaucoma. In some, this may occur with their very first attack and, in this state, there is no spontaneous resolution. The iris becomes jammed in the angle and any attempt at pupillary constriction will fail to remove the blockage.

The intraocular pressure will continue to rise and may reach 70 mmHg, a level at which a compensatory increase of ocular blood pressure is no longer possible. Consequently the eye will start to show internal ischaemic changes and eventually become externally congested. The symptoms of the acute attack are severe, with the water-logged cornea profoundly reducing the vision, and the eye becoming very painful. Nausea and vomiting may occur and the patient may even show physical shock.

The importance of early recognition and relief is paramount. The extremely high pressure can eventually cause optic atrophy of the ischaemic type, with or without cupping. The longer the attack persists, the poorer the prospect for full visual recovery.

Diagnosis

A subacute attack may be suspected from the patient's history but since the pressure may be normal between attacks diagnosis is difficult unless the patient is seen during an attack and the ocular pressure is measured. However, if the patient's symptoms are suggestive, the possibility of closed angle glaucoma should be considered, and suspicion should be further aroused if the anterior chamber is shallow, particularly if there is a family history of the condition.

The diagnosis can also be helped by an inspection of the angle of the anterior chamber with the gonioscope (see Figure 13.14). It will be found that the angle is narrow and the iris is close to the edge of the cornea, which contains

the canal of Schlemm, making it impossible to visualize the structures in the angle. Gonioscopy has an important negative value. If the angle appears unquestionably open at the time the eye pressure is elevated, the diagnosis of closed angle glaucoma can be excluded.

Confirmation of the diagnosis may be achieved by provoking an attack. The patient is placed in a dark environment (the 'dark room test'), or the pupil is dilated with drugs in a situation where this may be easily reversed by miotic drops. Either of these may cause a marked rise in the measured eye pressure. Alternatively, a therapeutic trial of pilocarpine drops may prove helpful. The symptoms of the subacute attack should be abolished within an hour of inserting the eyedrops.

An acute attack of closed angle glaucoma is recognizable from the following features, even without measurement of the intraocular pressure:

● Any painful, red eye with defective vision showing a characteristic, semi-dilated fixed pupil

● The pupil and iris are not clearly visible, the pupil appearing dark grey rather than black owing to the hazy cornea

● The eye is palpably hard, as is obvious, even on simple digital tonometry (see Figure 3.5).

Treatment

The pupil must be constricted in order to unblock the angle. The prime treatment is therefore to administer miotic drugs.

● Pilocarpine (usually 4 per cent) should be given intensively every five minutes for half an hour and every half an hour for two hours, and after that four times daily. The fellow eye, with its similar shallow anterior chamber, should also be given pilocarpine drops, four times daily, to prevent an attack occurring on that side.

● Acetazolamide should be given orally, or parenterally, as appropriate—500 mg immediately and 250 mg four times daily.

● Osmotic agents such as intravenous mannitol or oral glycerol may be needed. These reduce the intraocular pressure nonspecifically, but the effect is of course only temporary, lasting no more than a few hours.

● Analgesia is essential. Pethidine (100 mg) is appropriate in severe cases, and is given by injection if vomiting precludes oral administration.

Surgery

Peripheral iridectomy is indicated once the intraocular pressure has been reduced by the treatment outlined above. This can be done by surgery or by laser, and its purpose is to allow communication between the posterior and anterior chambers so the aqueous humour can bypass the pupil. A hole is made in the iris which prevents the accumulation of aqueous humour causing the periphery of the iris to bulge. Thus when the pupil dilates, the iris cannot close the angle (Figures 13.18 and 13.19).

The surgery is simple and is carried out not only on the affected eye, but prophylactically on the fellow eye; if the continued constriction of the pupil in the fellow eye is not maintained with pilocarpine drops, the risk of developing closed angle glaucoma, subacute or acute, is always present.

Various laser techniques are also available to produce a hole in the periphery of the iris without the necessity for formal surgery. However, some cases are not suitable for this.

As in chronic simple glaucoma, surgery for the closed angle type may be only partly successful. Medical treatment and even further surgery may be necessary postoperatively.

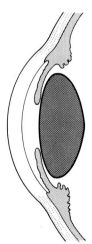
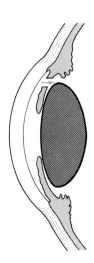
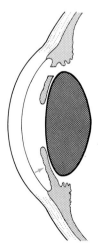
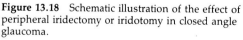

Figure 13.18 Schematic illustration of the effect of peripheral iridectomy or iridotomy in closed angle glaucoma.

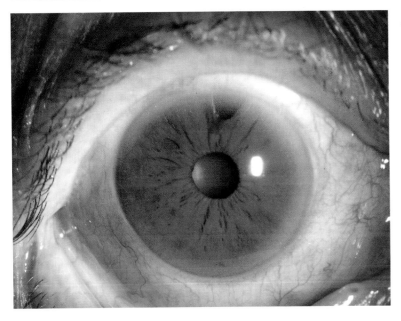

Figure 13.19 A peripheral iridectomy.

Prognosis of closed angle glaucoma

It is possible to maintain a patient with closed angle glaucoma on miotic drugs indefinitely, but this is not a guarantee against further attacks.

● **Subacute closed angle glaucoma**   Surgery will arrest the recurrence of subacute attacks of this condition, and if there has been no cumulative damage to the optic nerve during the repeated attacks, then the outlook for preservation of sight is very good.

● **Acute closed angle glaucoma**   A satisfactory outcome will depend on early diagnosis and rapid treatment, especially in the patient with an acute red eye. Apart from the effect of a continued high pressure on the optic nerve, any delay in the management of the condition predisposes the patient to cataract when the intraocular pressure has been returned to normal.

PRACTICAL POINTS

● Chronic simple glaucoma may go unnoticed by the patient if it affects only the peripheral field.

● Diagnosis is by measurement of pressures, inspection of the fundus for cupping of the optic disc and charting of the visual fields.

● Loss of visual function from chronic simple glaucoma is permanent and may possibly be prevented by the routine measurement of eye pressures in middle life. This is especially so in patients at particular risk from the disease, for example, those who have a family history. Such patients should be periodically observed.

● In established cases, continued medical treatment is required. If this does not control the pressure, laser therapy or drainage surgery is indicated.

● Subacute closed angle glaucoma occurs in attacks characterized by coloured rings, haloes around lights, pain and misty vision. Such an attack may resolve spontaneously or may progress to the acute stage. This requires immediate treatment to prevent the possibility of optic atrophy.

● Surgery or laser treatment can successfully prevent the recurrence of subacute attacks, and is mandatory after acute closed angle glaucoma has been brought under control by medical treatment.

● In patients with established closed angle glaucoma in one eye, surgery or laser iridectomy is advisable on the possibly unaffected fellow eye.

14   The conjunctiva and conjunctivitis

The conjunctiva is a thin, sparsely vascularized, transparent membrane which covers and protects the sclera, and forms the inner lining of the eyelids.

● **The bulbar conjunctiva** lies loosely over the eye so as not to restrict eye movement. It is firmly attached to the globe only at the corneoscleral junction.

● **The tarsal conjunctiva** lines the inner surface of the eyelids, to which it firmly adheres.

The bulbar and tarsal conjunctivae are continuous with each other at the upper and lower fornices. The conjunctiva ends at the lid margin where it becomes continuous with the skin of the eyelids.

The white sclera is visible through the conjunctiva, although some loose connective tissue (the episclera) actually separates the two. Also separating them are the front ends of the rectus muscles, covered by their own muscle sheaths, and the connective tissue layer known as Tenon's capsule.

In opththalmological textbooks, it is customary to describe the cornea and conjunctiva in close association, and there is no denying that some cases of conjunctival inflammation are complicated by corneal involvement. In this book, the placing of conjunctiva as part of the ophthalmic

protective mechanism may appear provocative, but this is done deliberately to emphasize the fact that the conjunctiva is not part of the visual apparatus. It should always be remembered that defective vision is not caused by conjunctival inflammation and, if in a case of conjunctivitis the vision is reduced, then there is some cause for it other than the conjunctivitis.

Conjunctival inflammation covers an important group of eye diseases. Acute infective conjunctivitis is the commonest cause of an acute red eye (see Chapter 3).

Infective conjunctivitis

Infective conjunctivitis may be caused by bacteria or smaller micro-organisms.

Bacterial conjunctivitis

In this condition the patient has a noticeable pink eye which is sticky, showing either obvious discharge or the eyelids being glued together after sleep (Figure 14.1). There is no pain, but a gritty, sandy feeling (even a foreign body sensation) is a common complaint. The patient's sight is unaffected and the pupil size and reactions are normal. The redness of the eye is

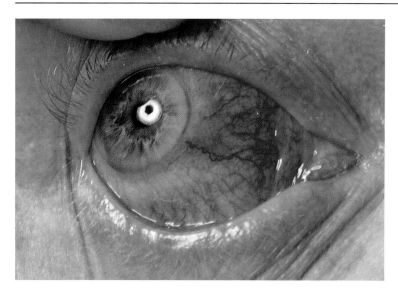

Figure 14.1 Bacterial conjunctivitis. Most of the redness is away from the cornea.

diffusely distributed. Although it starts on one side, the other eye may be involved quite quickly. The organisms usually responsible for bacterial conjunctivitis are staphylococci, pneumococci and the haemophilus group.

Investigation and treatment are often simple, the condition responding rapidly to antibiotic drops such as chloramphenicol or neomycin, inserted hourly for two to three days. The affected eye should not be covered. Cultures are not normally worth taking, unless ophthalmia neonatorum (the name given to conjunctivitis in the newborn) is suspected.

Strict personal hygiene is advisable for all patients suffering from bacterial conjunctivitis because it is common for whole families to be rapidly affected.

Acute conjunctivitis should always prompt inspection of the eyelids for blepharitis, entropion and ectropion (see pages 153–9), all of which may predispose to the condition.

Viral conjunctivitis

This common condition presents slightly differently from other types of conjunctivitis. In addition to the signs that occur in bacterial conjunctivitis, a follicular reaction is common in the tarsal surface of the upper lid, which may become heavy and half-shut (Figure 14.2). Preauricular lymph gland enlargement may sometimes occur.

All cases of virus conjunctivitis may be followed by corneal involvement. If this should

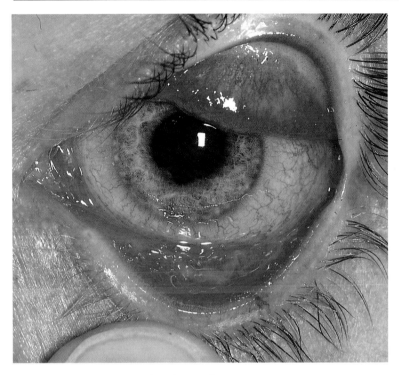

Figure 14.2 Viral conjuctivitis. The tarsal conjunctiva shows a follicular reaction.

occur, the patient may become photophobic and any discharge present will become watery. The cornea may show scattered punctate erosions, or infiltrates, and deep inflammation sometimes develops. In order to identify the corneal changes, a slit-lamp examination is necessary.

Investigation and treatment   Many viruses may be responsible for viral conjunctivitis. Herpes simplex, the adenoviruses and picorna viruses are common agents. Identifying the type of virus present can take some time, often a matter of weeks, and specific antiviral agents may not be available. Though a range of antiherpes simplex agents are now available, these are usually reserved for obvious corneal complication such as a dendritic ulcer (see Chapter 8).

Most cases of viral conjunctivitis resolve with or without treatment, but it is not unusual for the patient to suffer severe discomfort for two to three weeks. A chronically irritable eye may persist for several months.

The use of steroids in the management of viral conjunctivitis is in dispute. For example, if they are given to a patient with unsuspected herpes simplex, then keratitis may develop and run rampant: a dendritic ulcer may form and spread irregularly in an eye which is apparently whitening owing to a general anti-inflammatory action of steroids. It is for these reasons that a slit-lamp examination should always be carried out. If a slit-lamp is not available, then steroids must be avoided if there is any sign of corneal fluorescein staining. The only exception is when local steroid treatment is given under an ophthalmologist's supervision. In many cases, steroids do alleviate the signs and discomfort of virus conjunctivitis.

The chlamydia

The chlamydia are important ocular infective agents which produce conjunctival intracellular inclusions. The diseases they cause are known as 'tric' infections, the term being an acronym derived from **tr**achoma and **in**clusion **c**onjunctivitis.

Trachoma is an infective conjunctivitis, which is endemic in many underdeveloped countries and probably remains the commonest cause of blindness worldwide. It typically starts as follicular conjunctivitis, often acute, of the upper tarsal conjunctiva, later involving the conjunctiva of the eyeball, the cornea and the lid substance. The cornea becomes infiltrated by granulation tissue growing from above (pannus), which distorts and reduces vision (Figures 14.3 and 14.4). The cornea and the lid margins may become ulcerated, especially if secondary bacterial infection supervenes. The eyelashes may be destroyed or become misdirected, possibly initiating or aggravating corneal ulceration. In advanced cases, dense corneal scarring can seriously affect the vision. Perforation of the cornea and intraocular infection may also occur.

Trachoma is now fortunately becoming less widespread as the general environmental conditions in developing countries improve. The sensitivity of chlamydia to chemotherapy has also been an important factor in reducing the incidence.

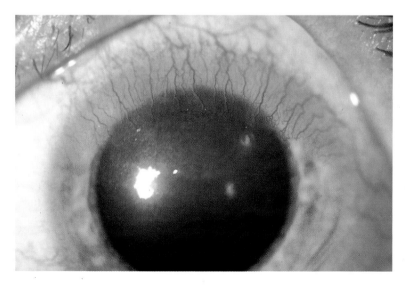

Figure 14.3   Infiltration of the upper cornea with new vessels in a case of trachoma.

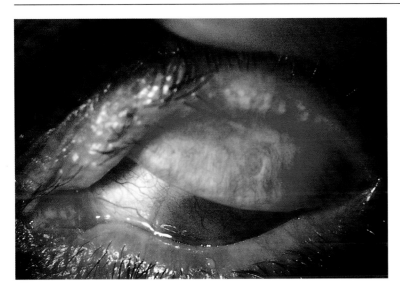

Figure 14.4 The late stage of trachoma and its effect on the eyelids The edge of the lid is distorted in shape and the eyelashes are turning back to abrade the cornea.

Inclusion conjunctivitis is the form that chlamydial infection takes in Western society. The chlamydia may be of a different strain from that of trachoma and produce a low-grade follicular conjunctivitis with associated corneal involvement similar to that produced by other virus infections. Numerous infiltrates occur. At one time the infection was known as 'swimming-bath conjunctivitis'. In certain cases the condition is venereally transmitted, and the chlamydia are responsible for a proportion of cases of cervicitis and urethritis. In addition, the organism may be a cause of ophthalmia neonatorum found in the newborn.

Investigation and treatment Chlamydial infections are identifiable by the presence of typical inclusion bodies found in the conjunctival cells obtained from scrapings of the tarsal surface of the eyelid and by culture of the organism from swabs of the conjunctiva.

Many cases of trachoma do not progress far, even without treatment. After the initial acute conjunctivitis, the chronic stage diminishes in most subjects to leave only a slight scarring of the tarsal surface of the lid and perhaps a minute infiltration of the upper cornea, which has no permanent effect on the vision.

It is in only a minority, none the less a significant one, that the condition proceeds to the severe degree described above.

Vigorous treatment of all chlamydial infections must include tetracyclines, sulphonamides or erythromycin, given locally and systemically. Typically, oxytetracycline would be given by mouth, 250 mg three or four times daily for three weeks. The distortion of the eyelids and eyelashes, which are a feature of advanced trachoma, may necessitate minor to even extensive plastic surgery of the eyelids.

Non-infective conjunctivitis

Non-infective conjunctivitis embraces many possible causes: allergic, chemical or physical.

Allergic conjunctivitis

The condition may be associated with lid allergies. It also occurs commonly in hayfever. Itching is a distinct complaint in this type of inflammation.

One form that may be associated with a general allergic diathesis is the so-called 'spring catarrh', which is characterized by photophobia and a watery, stringy discharge. Some corneal irritation is always present, perhaps associated with large cobblestone papillae which are often found under the upper lid (Figure 14.5). Steroids may be indicated, but sodium cromoglycate should be used first (see Chapter 21).

Many cases of allergic conjunctivitis are chronic or recurrent. The continuous suppressive or active use of steroids may lead to an unsuspected glaucoma. For this reason, all patients on this therapy for whatever condition should have regular checks taken of their intraocular pressure.

Physical and chemical conjunctivitis

The condition is more accurately termed 'chronic conjunctival hyperaemia'. Some of the factors

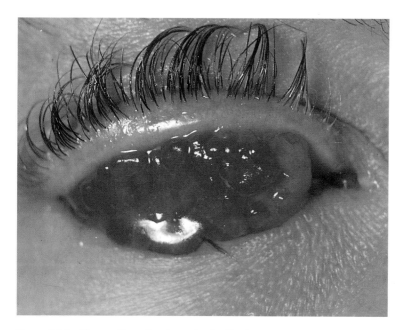

Figure 14.5   The papillae of spring catarrh affecting the conjuctiva.

responsible for the condition are windy or dusty environments, excessive light, industrial chemicals, as well as some cosmetics and alcohol and nicotine abuse. In these cases, astringent drops (zinc preparations), vasoconstrictors (adrenaline), antihistamines and local antibiotics and steroids (often in varying combinations) may be dispensed. The treatment may often appear less rational than the obvious remedy of withdrawal of the physical or chemical agent responsible. This, however, is a counsel of perfection in many cases as the offending agent, whether physical, chemical or allergic, may be impossible to identify or remove.

Chronic conjunctivitis

The symptoms of chronic conjunctivitis, usually without grossly abnormal signs, are common clinical problems presented to the family physician:

- General irritation and occasional redness of the eyes

- Hot, burning or dry eyes

- Foreign body sensation.

The clinical picture is sometimes part of 'eyestrain' (see Chapter 4). Once the causes of eyestrain are eliminated, an examination of the eye will show it to be relatively uninflamed with no lid, corneal or pupillary signs, with normal tear flow and no general or local skin condition. It is often impossible to diagnose a particular organic cause.

Investigation and treatment Conjunctival swabs may be taken to eliminate an infective

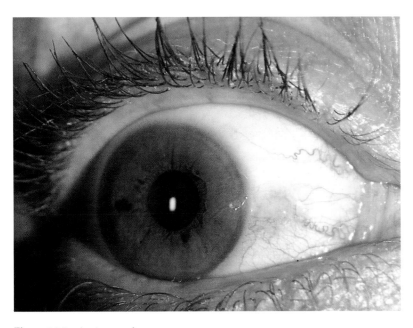

Figure 14.6   A pingueculum.

cause. Deficient tear production should be eliminated. Recourse is often made to the remedies mentioned above for physical or chemical conjunctivitis (see page 134). Even if the condition responds to treatment, this may simply be a placebo effect. In many instances this group of symptoms is psychogenic in origin.

Other conjunctival conditions

Serious conjunctival conditions, for example, tumours, are uncommon. Where lesions such as malignant melanomata do occur, they may be treated by the radiotherapist with strontium 90.

Penetration should be limited so that radiation cataract does not occur.

Degenerative changes do occur quite frequently, and these can give rise to anxiety on cosmetic grounds. Typical of these is pingueculum, which is an aging change that presents as a slightly yellowish patch of degeneration occurring in the area exposed between the lids, usually nasal to the cornea (Figure 14.6). This condition is often prominent when the eye is inflamed because the lesion itself is avascular. It is best left alone. If cosmetic considerations are important, surgical excision is possible, but the condition may recur. Pingueculum should never be confused with pterygium (see page 69).

PRACTICAL POINTS

● Acute bacterial conjunctivitis is the commonest cause of a red eye. There is discharge and the pupil and vision are normal.

● Viral conjunctivitis differs from other types in having a more prolonged course and may be followed by corneal involvement.

● Blepharitis, ectropion and entropion predispose towards acute conjunctivitis.

● Steroids should be avoided as treatment for patients suspected of having viral conjunctivitis, or where the diagnosis is uncertain. Referral for slit-lamp examination is advisable in these cases.

● Trachoma and chlamydial conjunctivitis are now far less common in developing countries owing to improved hygiene and successful chemotherapy. In Western society, chlamydia often presents as a recalcitrant conjunctivitis.

● Patients with allergic conjunctivitis being treated with steroids should be monitored for glaucoma.

● 'Chronic conjunctivitis' is a vague group of conditions, physical, chemical or psychogenic in origin. Placebos are often prescribed in the absence of clear therapeutic indications.

● Pingueculum, which should not be confused with pterygium, is best left untreated.

15   Wet and dry eyes

The lacrimal apparatus is an important part of the ocular protective system. The tears are nutritional to the cornea and keep it moist, so preventing the development of dry areas which could become ulcerated or secondarily infected. The tears also lubricate the movement of the eyelids over the eyeball. Their origin is in the lacrimal gland, the ducts of which enter the upper, outer region of the conjunctival sac and drain into the lacrimal puncta in the inner part of the lid margins. This cross-flow prevents any atmospheric debris from lodging in the cornea or conjunctiva. The flow is reflexly increased as a result of any possible, harmful stimulae or inflammation of the front of the eye.

From the lacrimal puncta tears drain via the canaliculi, lacrimal sac and nasolacrimal duct into the inferior meatus of the nose (Figure 15.1).

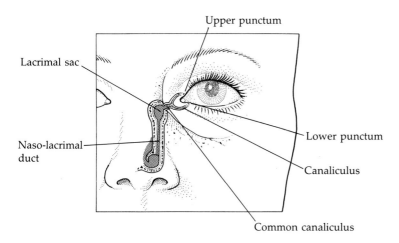

Figure 15.1   The lacrimal drainage system.

WATERING EYES

Eyes water for one of two reasons:

- The tear drainage is defective (epiphora).

- Excessive tears are produced (lacrimation).

Epiphora

As an isolated clinical complaint, watering of the eyes is usually due to defective drainage and occurs principally at two periods of life:

1 During infancy when the lower end of the nasolacrimal duct is imperforate due to incomplete canalization

2 During middle life when the duct or other parts of the drainage pathway may be organically or functionally obstructed. The watering is often aggravated in windy or cold weather conditions.

The watering eye during infancy In infants, not only may one or both eyes water, but often there is some discharge owing to stasis and secondary infection of the tears in the lacrimal sac. Treatment consists of applying pressure over the sac (Figure 15.2). This 'expression', if carried out regularly for some weeks (three or four times daily) and followed by drops of an appropriate antibiotic, such as chloramphenicol, may blow open the entry of the nasolacrimal duct into the nose. In many cases the condition resolves itself even without treatment, but if this regime fails then the tear passages should be probed under general anaesthesia. Unless the stickiness and watering are extreme, probing is best delayed until after the infant's first birthday.

The watering eye in adults This should be investigated by syringing of the tear ducts (Figure 15.3) and, if indicated, by dacryocystography (Figure 15.4).

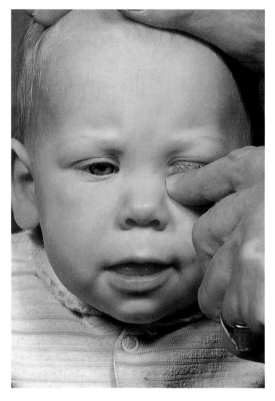

Figure 15.2 Expression of the lacrimal sac. Pressure is exerted downwards and backwards through the lower eyelid, between the lower inner orbital margin and the eyeball.

Unfortunately, a high proportion of adults suffering from watering eyes do not show any significant obstruction. The watering often seems to be a functional stasis due perhaps to a laxity of that part of the orbicularis oculi which surrounds the lacrimal sac and which normally pumps the tears away (the 'lacrimal pump'). Helpful measures for this so-called 'symptomatic epiphora' are limited. For example, astringent drops (zinc sulphate combined with adrenaline) may shrink up a supposedly congested lacrimal

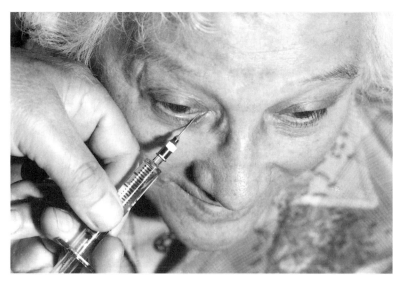

Figure 15.3 Syringing of the tear ducts.

mucosa, and direct surgery on the lacrimal gland may occasionally be helpful.

The common sites of organic lacrimal obstructions are illustrated in Figure 15.1.

Eversion of the lower lacrimal punctum may be found either alone or as part of ectropion (see page 160). The eversion may be reduced or abolished by cauterization of the conjunctiva below the punctum.

Investigation may reveal that the obstruction is in the canaliculi, the lacrimal sac, or in the nasolacrimal duct.

All the major forms of lacrimal obstruction may require the re-establishment of tear drainage into the nose by the operation of dacryocystorhinostomy (DCR). In this procedure the lining of the lacrimal sac is anastomosed to the nasal mucosa of the middle meatus after removing the intervening bone. Fine plastic tubes may be left temporarily, or permanently, in the anastomosis to preserve its patency.

In the adult, as in the infant, obstruction of the tear flow downstream from the lacrimal sac can lead to a secondary infection of the tears in the sac itself. This may be chronic and there may be a quiet intermittent regurgitation of mucoid or purulent material into the conjunctival sac, with a variable swelling, a mucocoele, visible over the site of the lacrimal sac itself (Figure 15.5). The swelling can often be reduced in size by simple exertion of external pressure on it.

Occasionally, acute infection supervenes and leads to acute dacryocystitis, producing a swollen, inflamed, painful, tender area (Figure 15.6). This is treated by local and systemic chemotherapy and, if appropriate, by surgical drainage.

Lacrimation

Primary excessive tear production as a cause of eye watering appears to be uncommon.

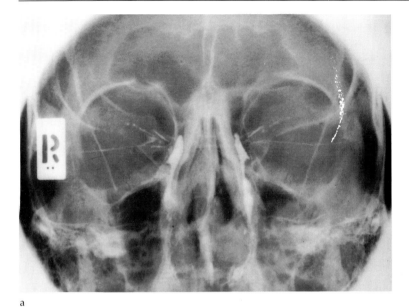

a

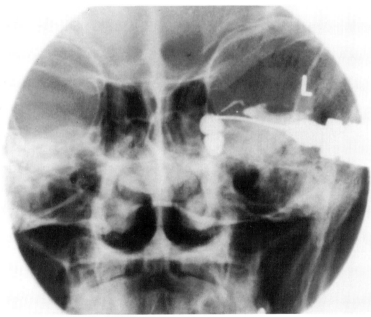

b

Figure 15.4 Dacryocystograms: (*a*) shows a normal
tear drainage system on both sides. The radio opaque
fluid passes down from the tear sacs through the
nasolacrimal ducts to the pharynx. (*b*) shows an
obstructed nasolacrimal duct with an enlarged bifid
lacrimal sac.

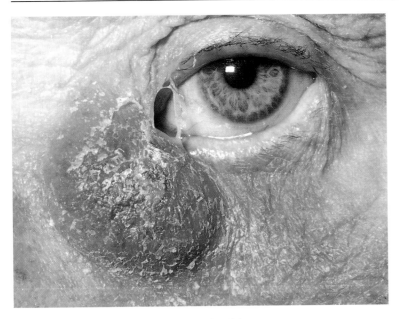

Figure 15.5   A recently infected mucocoele of the lacrimal sac.

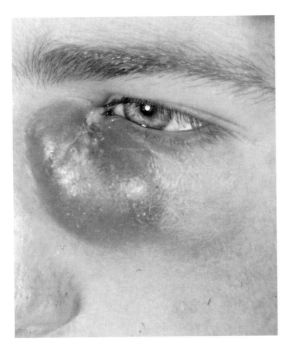

Figure 15.6   Acute dacryocystitis.

Secondary lacrimation is very frequent as a result of inflammatory conditions of the outer segment of the globe. These include corneal irritation, resulting from ulceration or caused by a foreign body, iritis and acute closed angle glaucoma.

Lacrimation is also a marked feature of allergic conditions affecting the outer eye, with or without simultaneous involvement of the nasal mucosa.

DRY EYES

The common complaint of dry eyes is rarely confirmed by the actual measurement of the tear flow, or by inspection of the eyes; it is occasionally simply a symptom of chronic conjunctival inflammation, whether bacterial or environmental, although more usually this condition leads to the opposite complaint of eye watering.

Dryness of the eyes is often given as an explanation, on somewhat dubious grounds, for some difficulty experienced in wearing or adapting to contact lenses.

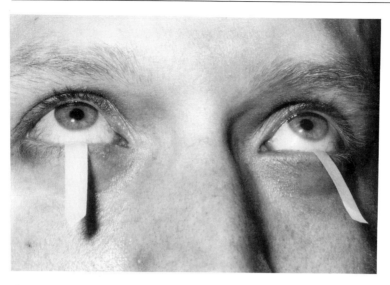

Figure 15.7   The Schirmer filter paper test for estimating the volume of lacrimal secretion. Standardized papers are left in place for five minutes. A normal tear flow wets them to some 15 mm down from the lid margins.

True defective tear production occurs in Sjögren's syndrome where atrophy of the lacrimal gland occurs and the dryness leads to a filamentary necrosis of the corneal epithelium. Patients with this condition have very uncomfortable, congested and often photophobic eyes.

Rheumatoid arthritis is the most frequent association of the Sjögren picture. The condition may have an autoimmune basis, as it is sometimes found in other collagen diseases as well as primary biliary cirrhosis. In sarcoidosis, lacrimal gland enlargement may occur but there may also be a deficiency of tear production.

Dry eyes, with deficiency of tear production confirmed by the Schirmer test (Figure 15.7), need frequent applications of drops such as normal saline, Ringer-Locke solution or hypromellose (methylcellulose), or more complex formulations which have polyvinyl alcohol in them, if the simpler remedies fail to help. For no very clear reason, it has been found that some patients are helped by the sealing of the lacrimal puncta.

PRACTICAL POINTS

● Watering eyes are classified as epiphora, defective tear drainage or lacrimation, or excessive tear production. These are common conditions in infancy or middle life.

● In infancy, the tear sac should be expressed by external pressure. Should a watering, sticky eye persist, probing is the means of opening the nasolacrimal duct, but this is best avoided in infants under one year of age.

● There appears to be no organic obstruction of the tear ducts in many adults complaining of epiphora.

● Surgical treatment may be indicated if a site of obstruction can be identified.

● Tears retained in the lacrimal sac may be secondarily infected, leading to acute dacrocystitis or to a more chronic condition of a mucocoele.

● Lacrimation can be a symptom of various inflammatory or allergic conditions.

● Rheumatoid arthritis is the most common disease associated with true defective tear production.

16   Prominent and not so prominent eyes

An eye may appear conspicuous for any of the following three reasons:

- It may actually be large, though this is rare

- A normal sized eye may appear large because it is pushed forward, proptosed

- The palpebral aperture of the normal sized eye may be wide, for example, when upper lid retraction is present.

PROPTOSIS

The term exophthalmos is often used interchangeably for proptosis (Figure 16.1). The most common cause of bilateral proptosis and, incidentally, also of unilateral proptosis, is dysthyroid disease. This is discussed further in Chapter 25.

All other causes of proptosis are rare, but include vascular malformations of the orbit, such as cavernous haemangioma, lacrimal gland swellings and mucocoeles of the frontal or ethmoidal sinuses. There is also a rare and ill-defined entity of pseudotumour of the orbit which appears to be a granulomatous affection.

Malignancies, either secondary or of primary orbital structures, are also uncommon; those that are more frequently encountered usually arise in the lacrimal glands or the paranasal sinuses. In children, primary rhabdomyosarcoma and secondary deposits from the adrenals are occasionally encountered.

Symptoms and signs

Proptosis is often symptomless, but the patient may feel there is a cosmetic disability and is sometimes told he has a 'stare'. Exposure may give rise to mild conjunctival hyperaemia and a true corneal involvement may present as an acute red eye (see Chapter 3). The forward position of the cornea allows it to dry, making it susceptible to ulceration and secondary infection. The situation may be aggravated if the lids do not close fully over the front of the globe, especially if there is also upper lid retraction and particularly during sleep.

The early sign of such a problem is some fine fluorescein punctate staining of the lower third of the cornea. Some cases may proceed to ulceration or abrasion, and secondary infection with the rare but very serious consequences of perforation and intraocular sepsis.

This is one threat to the sight; it may also be at risk due to compression of the optic nerve by the agent pushing the eye forward.

As displacement of the globe will also interfere with the action of the ocular muscles, perhaps

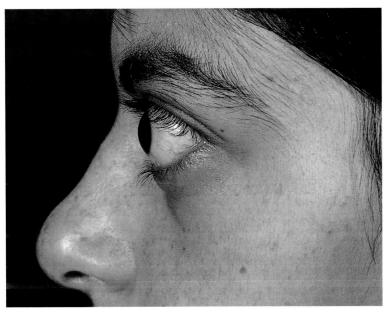

Figure 16.1 A proptosed eye.

giving rise to diplopia, the ocular movements should be examined in all cases of proptosis.

Degree and type of proptosis

Examination for minimal degrees of proptosis is best carried out as illustrated in Figures 16.2 and 16.3. A common mistake is to identify an eye with a slight degree of ectropion of the lower lid as being proptosed. In true proptosis, the sclera may be visible above, as well as below, the cornea. If the sclera is visible only above the cornea, the condition may turn out to be simply lid retraction which can be present without true proptosis.

Follow-up of an established proptosis is by serial measurement using a proptometer (Figure 16.4).

The direction of displacement of the eyeball is also important and may indicate the origin of the condition. A lacrimal gland swelling will, for example, not only push the eye forwards but also downwards and inwards. Swellings of paranasal origin displace the eye outwards as well as forwards (see Figure 16.5).

Diagnosis and treatment

Although the diagnosis of the cause of proptosis, and its treatment, may be complex, the ophthalmologist is particularly concerned at an early stage to ensure that the health of the cornea is satisfactory. If this is the case, and if the condition remains stable with an identified benign cause, no action is indicated provided

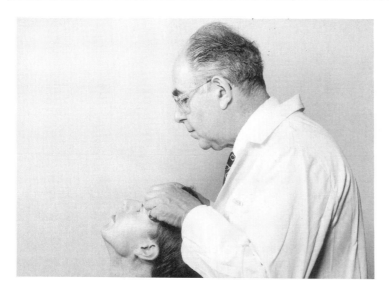

Figure 16.2   Inspecting the eyes from above for
proptosis.

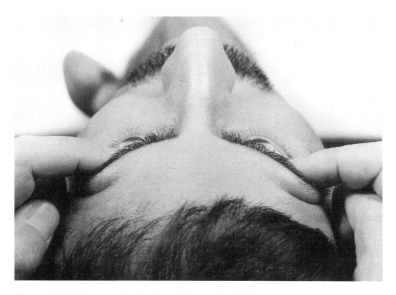

Figure 16.3   The examiner's view. The patient looks
downwards and the examiner approaches from behind
to see which cornea appears first.

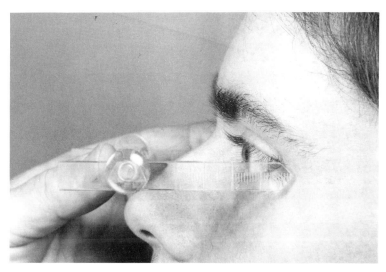

Figure 16.4   A simple instrumental method of measuring proptosis.

the patient is not troubled by the cosmetic appearance.

Simple measures, lubricant, astringent vaso-constrictor drops and various forms of tarsorr-haphy may be indicated if there is evidence of corneal exposure. Lateral tarsorrhaphy may, in any event, be indicated purely for cosmetic purposes. Central tarsorrhaphy may be manda-tory if serious corneal ulceration has developed (see Chapter 17).

In diagnosis, CT scanning and, in some cases, ultrasound have made a considerable impact (Figures 16.5 and 16.6). Surgical exploration of the orbit may still be necessary to determine the cause and can be a therapeutic procedure if the investigation, or the procedure itself, reveals that some removable tumour is the cause of the condition.

Orbital exploration may also ultimately be indicated in order to safeguard the eye itself. A decompression of the orbit may, for example, be required in extreme dysthyroid proptosis. This allows the contents of the orbit to expand beyond one of its bony walls, which is removed.

ENOPHTHALMOS

Enophthalmos is a condition where the eye has sunk back into its socket. It is much rarer than

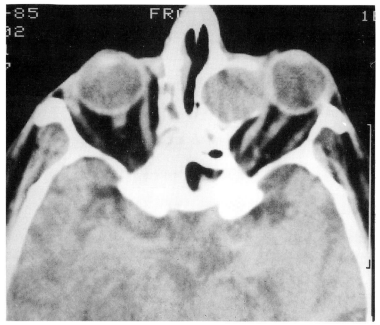

Figure 16.5   A CT scan of both orbits of a patient with
an ethmoidal mucocoele on the right side.

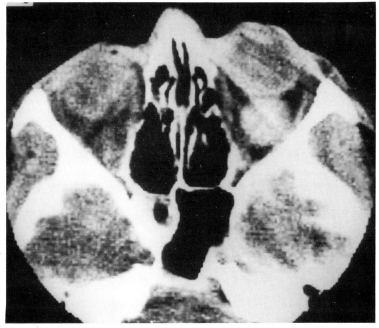

Figure 16.6   A CT scan of an orbital haemangioma
causing proptosis of the right eye.

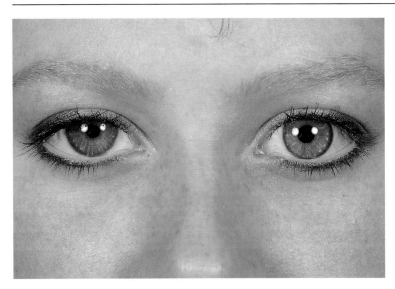

Figure 16.7 Horner's syndrome. The right pupil is slightly smaller than the left and there is ptosis of the right upper lid.

proptosis and may be falsely diagnosed if, for some reason, the fellow eye is unduly prominent. If the upper lid shows ptosis, the eye likewise appears to have receded when it has not actually done so. This last situation is believed to account for the enophthalmos of Horner's syndrome, sympathetic paralysis, and is associated with a relatively small pupil on the affected side (Figure 16.7). Otherwise the commonest cause of true enophthalmos is probably some form of trauma to the orbital bones (the 'blow-out fracture') (see Figure 18.8). Bilateral enophthalmos sometimes occurs in old age, owing to atrophy of orbital fat.

PRACTICAL POINTS

● The most common cause of protrusion of the eyeball, proptosis, is dysthyroid disease, and this is true whether the proptosis is bilateral, as is usual, or, less commonly, unilateral.

● Apart from the cosmetic problems associated with a staring eye, the main difficulty arises from the possible exposure of the cornea.

● There may also be abnormalities of the movements of the eyes and interference with optic nerve function, leading to loss of vision or of visual field.

● Enophthalmos, the opposite condition to proptosis, is perhaps most frequently the result of injury to the orbital bones.

17   The eyelids

The eyelids are covered by skin on the outside and conjunctiva on the inside. Between these lies a thick layer of tough fibrous tissue, the tarsal plate, which maintains the shape of the lid, keeping it approximated to the eye (Figure 17.1).

The eyelids close to protect the eyes in sleep and intermittently during blinking, either spontaneously, or in response to any external threat. During closure the upper lids move more than the lower. The edges of the lids are normally in contact during blinking and sleeping. In addition to giving mechanical protection to the eye, the movements of the lids encourage tears to flow across the cornea, thus keeping it moist.

The eyelids contain two opposing muscles, the orbicularis oculi, which is responsible for closure, innervated by the VIIth cranial nerve; and the levator palpebrae superioris, which keeps the eye open by lifting the upper lid. It is innervated by the IIIrd cranial nerve and by the sympathetic system, being partly voluntary and partly smooth muscle.

The meibomian glands, situated in the tarsal plate and opening on the edge of each eyelid, produce an oily secretion that mixes with the watery component of the tears. The secretion is believed to be important in preserving the health of the cornea. Lipid-producing and sweat glands open into the follicles of the eyelashes. The protective function of the eyelashes is primordial.

General skin conditions may affect the skin of the eyelids, and some conjunctival problems can involve the inner lid surface. Most abnormalities of eyelids fall into one of the following categories:

- Localized swellings
- Generalized swellings
- Age changes
- Abnormal lid positions
- Abnormal movements of the eyelids.

LOCALIZED SWELLINGS

These types of swellings may or may not be associated with inflammation.

Inflammatory swellings

These may be caused by, for example, a stye, an infection of an eyelash follicle, or by secondary infection of a meibomian cyst. The swelling is red, painful and tender (see Figure 3.9).

Antibiotic drops or ointments, three of four times daily, will normally resolve the condition with or without discharge of purulent contents. Local heat (hot spoon bathing) can be soothing.

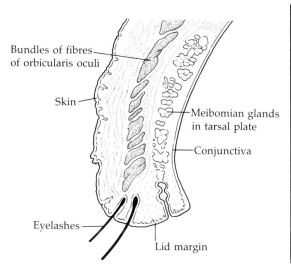

Bundles of fibres of orbicularis oculi

Skin

Meibomian glands in tarsal plate

Conjunctiva

Eyelashes

Lid margin

Figure 17.1   The anatomy of the eyelid.

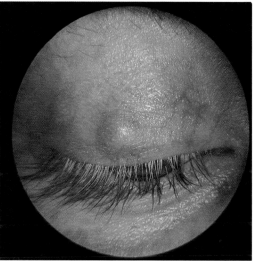

Figure 17.2   A meibomian cyst presenting externally.

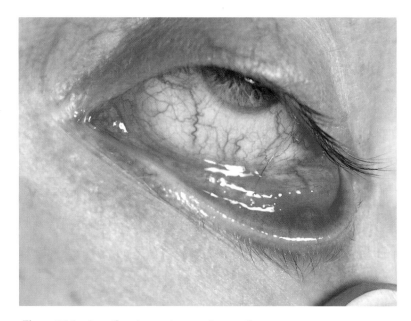

Figure 17.3   A meibomian cyst presenting on the conjunctival surface of the eyelid.

Non-inflammatory swellings

A meibomian cyst, or chalazion (Figure 17.2), is the commonest non-inflammatory swelling. It is a granulomatous response to retained secretion in one or more of the meibomian glands. The condition may present in a number of ways, two of which are illustrated (see also Figure 17.3).

Treatment is normally incision and scraping out of the contents, but if there is a thick wall brought about by a previous infection, excision may be necessary. The minor surgery is performed on the inside of the lid (the conjunctival aspect) so that there is no external scar. If the cyst is infected, surgery should be delayed until the infection has been eradicated by local chemotherapy.

Other cysts of the lid are frequently seen at the lid margin. These involve the lipid-producing glands and are recognized by the milky (Zeis' gland) or clear (Moll's gland) character of their contents (Figures 17.4 and 17.5). Tiny sebaceous cysts may occur anywhere on the skin surface of the lid. Simple cautery excision is adequate.

In the deeper substance of the lid, particularly at the outer part of the upper lid, dermoid cysts occur. These are congenital and contain dermal

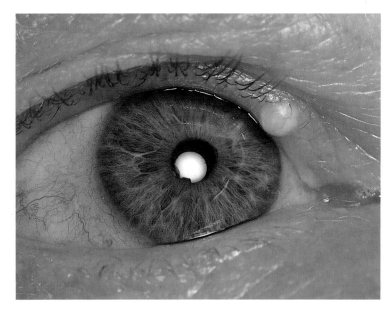

Figure 17.4   A cyst of Zeis's gland.

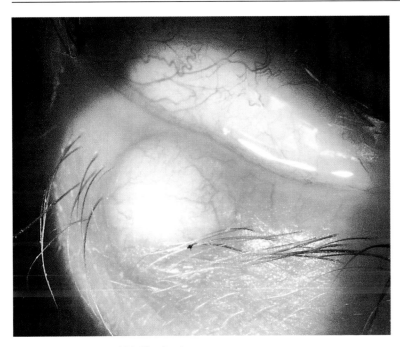

Figure 17.5   A cyst of Moll's gland.

and sebaceous material (Figure 17.6). They occasionally also involve the conjunctiva and cornea.

Tumours of the lid are not uncommon, typically papillomata and rodent ulcers, representing the benign and malignant type respectively (Figures 17.7 and 17.8). The former are treated by cautery excision, but the latter may be managed by surgery or radiotherapy. Surgery may involve wide excision, necessitating plastic reconstruction should there be a wide gap in the lid.

Lipid deposits (xanthelasma) are found especially in subjects with raised serum cholesterol

(Figure 17.9). They usually appear in the inner one-third of the eyelids, upper or lower. They are simple to excise, but may recur.

GENERALIZED SWELLINGS

These swellings include squamous blepharitis, allergic blepharitis and non-inflammatory oedema.

Squamous blepharitis

Typical findings in squamous blepharitis (Figure 17.10) are thickened red margins of the lids with

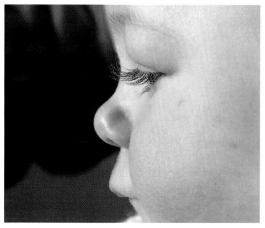

a

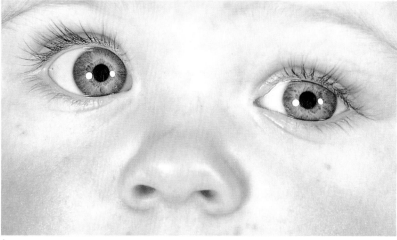

b

Figure 17.6 (*a*) and (*b*) A dermoid cyst of the outer angle of the eye in an infant.

white crusts in the roots of the lashes. The condition is very common and often constitutional. It is for this reason that anything other than a temporary abatement of treatment may be impossible to achieve. There is some association with seborrhoeic dermatitis, especially dandruff of the scalp. Secondary staphylococcal infection is common and predisposes to styes or infected chalazia.

Rosacea may be a background factor in some cases.

Management Local steroid treatment, perhaps combined with antibiotics, produces temporary

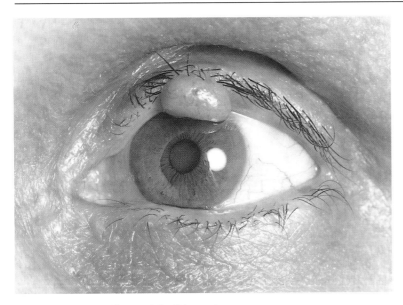

Figure 17.7   A papilloma of the lid margin.

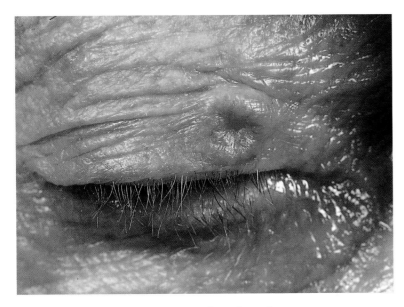

Figure 17.8   A basal cell carcinoma (rodent ulcer) of the right upper eyelid.

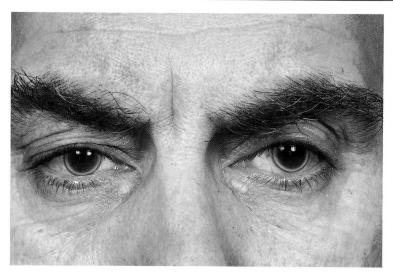

Figure 17.9   Xanthelasma.

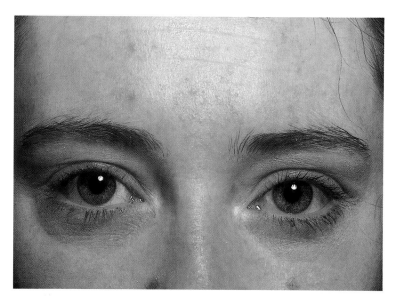

Figure 17.10   Mild blepharitis; the lid margins are quite pink.

improvement of the squamous blepharitis. Debridement of the scales accumulating in the roots of the eyelash can also be helpful; a simple lotion such as 3 per cent sodium bicarbonate may be used. Associated skin or scalp conditions should be treated.

Allergic blepharitis

In allergic blepharitis (Figure 17.11) there is an eczematous reaction of all the eyelid skin, not merely of the lid margins. The possible allergens responsible are set out below:

● Cosmetics are one of the main offenders, and not necessarily those applied directly to the eyelids; facial and more distant applications are also occasionally responsible.

● Eyedrops may cause allergic swelling of the lids, as well as allergic conjunctivitis. Of these, atropine, antibiotics such as neomycin and chloramphenicol and some drugs used in the treatment of glaucoma, are particularly prone to cause this type of swelling, especially when the drugs have been used for long periods of time.

● External allergens (plants, animals) can also give rise to general allergic lid swelling.

● Generalized allergic reactions, to systemically administered drugs, for example, involve the eyelids. The same applies to eyelids in subjects with the so-called 'allergic diathesis' or 'atopy', often a combination of asthma, hay fever and perhaps eczema.

Management   Identification and withdrawal of the allergen and local steroids are the usual

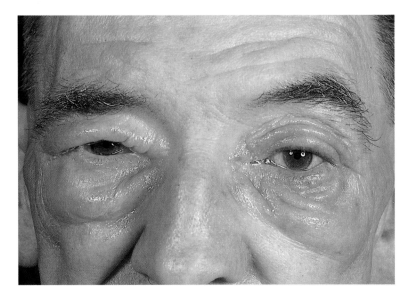

Figure 17.11   Allergic blepharitis due to sensitivity to eyedrops used for glaucoma.

management of allergic blepharitis. The dangers of prolonged use of steroids for eye conditions have been noted elsewhere (see page 122).

Non-inflammatory oedema

The eyelids are sometimes the site of the so-called fleeting 'angioneurotic oedema', which occurs in urticarial subjects. More persistent swellings may have an endocrine basis, typically dysthyroid, myxoedema affecting the lower lids, or the more widespread oedema of both the upper and lower lids, occurring with thyrotropic exophthalmos.

Oedema of the lids may also occur as part of a generalized oedema, as in renal disease.

Management   The management of these conditions is related to their systemic cause.

AGE CHANGES

Swelling of the lids associated with aging are frequent and often cosmetically distressing. The common bags under the eyes and the swelling in the inner upper lids are the result of a combination of decreasing skin elasticity and forward prolapse of the orbital fat, which is no longer restrained by the less taut orbital septum.

Management   Reassurance may be sufficient for many patients, but cosmetic plastic surgery is a possible alternative.

ABNORMAL POSITIONS OF THE LIDS AND EYELASHES

Entropion

In entropion the lid (Figure 17.12) rotates inwards so that the lid margin faces backwards

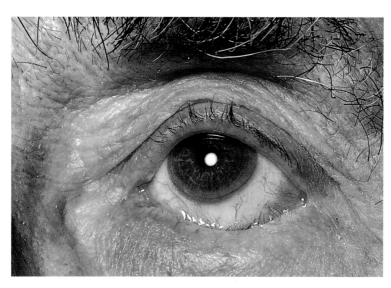

Figure 17.12   Spastic entropion. The condition often varies. At times the lid may look normal, but it can be induced to turn in by the patient screwing the eye up.

towards the eyeball. Although occasionally produced by scarring inside the lid from burns, the condition is usually what is termed spastic entropion of the lower lid, commonly occurring in later life. The precise cause is unknown. It seems, however, that where the marginal fibres of the orbicularis muscle approximate the two ends of the lower lid, the lid turns in and causes the eyelashes to abrade the conjunctiva and cornea. The patient consequently suffers from a very scratchy and uncomfortable eye. Temporary relief is obtained by rolling the eyelids outwards, using the finger, but the lid will immediately slip back to the inturned position.

Management Strapping applied to the lid to hold it out is only a preliminary to a minor surgical procedure, which should be performed to prevent the inward rotation. Unfortunately, spastic entropion has a habit of recurring and no surgical procedure has yet been devised to eliminate completely this possibility.

Ectropion

This is the opposite to entropion and again particularly affects the lower lid. In most cases the condition is due to senile atony of the orbicularis muscle, which can no longer prevent the dropping away of the eyelid. It also occurs as a regular feature of Bell's palsy or other types of facial paralysis (Figures 17.13 and 17.14).

The main effect of ectropion is to part the lower lacrimal punctum from the pool of tears so that the affected eye waters. This may lead to eczema, and the associated scarring and shrinkage of the skin aggravates the ectropion.

Management The exposure of the conjunctiva may lead to a secondary infection. The infection should be cleared up before minor surgery to tighten and, if appropriate, shorten the elongated and lax eyelid. Although the cosmetic improvement is relatively simple, successful repositioning of the lower lid and the lacrimal

punctum does not necessarily abolish the watering. This may be due to disuse atrophy of the other parts of the lacrimal drainage apparatus.

Trichiasis

Trichiasis is a misdirected eyelash abrading the cornea when the lid itself is in a normal position (Figure 17.15). This must be distinguished from entropion (see page 158).

Management Initially it is customary simply to pull out the offending eyelash or eyelashes. If they regrow in an abnormal direction, they can be removed permanently by electrolysis or cryotherapy.

Ptosis

This is dropping of the upper lid (Figure 17.16). Ptosis is usually due to a weakening of either the voluntary part or of the sympathetically innervated fibres of the levator palpebral superioris muscle.

In a child, ptosis is usually congenital and in some cases there is a definite hereditary factor. The condition is caused by a general weakness of the levator and may be associated with weakness of elevation of the eye. It is usually unilateral, occasionally bilateral. In a minority of cases, the cause appears to be misdirected innovation and the ptosis is much reduced when the mouth is opened, producing the effect known as 'jaw winking' during chewing.

In later life, acquired ptosis may indicate a IIIrd (oculomotor) nerve palsy or a sympathetic nerve deficiency (Horner's syndrome). A IIIrd nerve palsy may lead to diplopia, with obvious defects in eye movement. The pupil may be large in IIIrd nerve palsy, or small in Horner's syndrome.

Ptosis may be intermittent or variable, and this is a particular feature of the myopathic condition, myasthenia gravis.

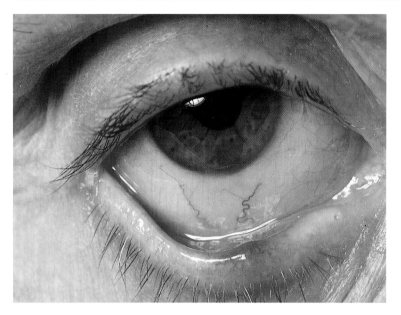

Figure 17.13 Mild ectropion of the lower lid.

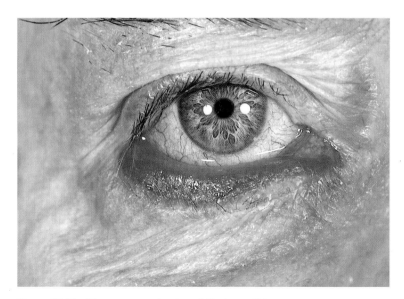

Figure 17.14 More severe ectropion of the lower lid.

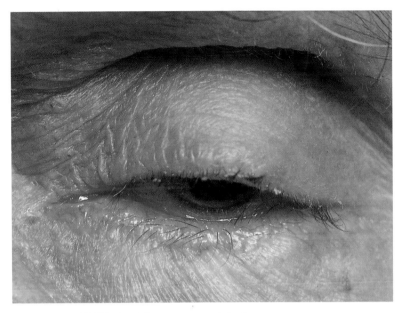

Figure 17.15   Trichiasis of the outer part of the lower lid.

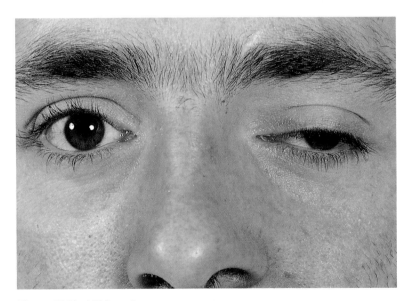

Figure 17.16   Mild ptosis.

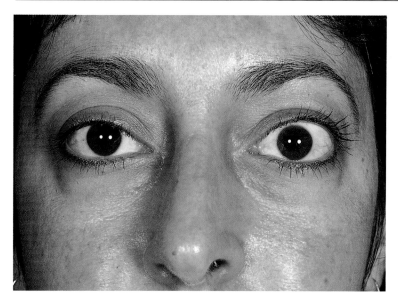

Figure 17.17   Lid retraction of the left eye.

Management   In childhood, operative treatment is indicated for cosmetic reasons, or if the pupil is significantly covered.

Lid retraction

This is a drawing back of the upper lid. Almost invariably a dysthyroid phenomenon, it aggravates the staring appearance produced by the associated proptosis (Figure 17.17).

Lagophthalmos

Lagophthalmos is the inability to close the eye (Figure 17.18). It is often caused by a VIIth nerve malfunction, Bell's palsy. Any degree of proptosis, whether dysthyroid or not, may also interfere with lid closure. The condition occasionally occurs in patients with scarred lids that simply cannot close, or in myopathic disorders.

A degree of lagophthalmos is often found in the deeply unconscious patient and is sometimes seen in normal subjects during sleep.

Whatever the cause, the condition may lead to exposure of the cornea, especially if associated with a poor 'Bell's phenomenon', which is upward rotation of the eye on attempted closure. Significant exposure will be indicated by fluorescein staining, typically of the lower third of the cornea.

Management   If the lagophthalmos is slight, the cornea may show no ill-effects and no action other than ordering some prophylactic or lubricant eyedrops is necessary. If the condition is

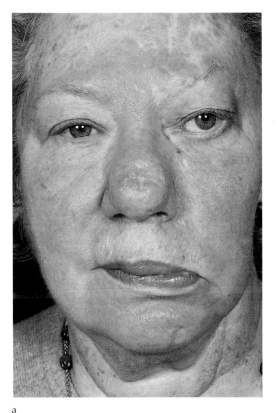 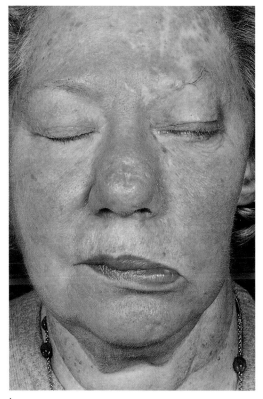

a   b

Figure 17.18 (*a*) and (*b*) Lagophthalmos–a case of old facial palsy on the left side. Note that on attempted closure (*b*), the lids do not meet. There is scarring of the forehead due to previous herpes zoster.

more severe, artificial lid closure may be needed, either by temporary strapping or by first denuding (to assist fusion) and then suturing the upper and lower eyelid margins together; a procedure called tarsorrhaphy (Figure 17.19). Surgical closure at the outer angle (lateral tarsorrhaphy) may be adequate but where severe corneal exposure and ulceration have already occurred, then closure of the lids, centrally, is necessary (central tarsorrhaphy). This cuts out the vision, but the tarsorrhaphy can be opened once the cornea has healed, provided the predisposing condition has abated, even if incompletely.

A protective soft contact lens is helpful where severe lagophthalmos has occurred and the lids cannot be closed, even surgically.

ABNORMAL MOVEMENTS OF THE EYELIDS

Abnormal movements of the eyelids often take the form of a localized myokymia and spasmodic closure of the lids.

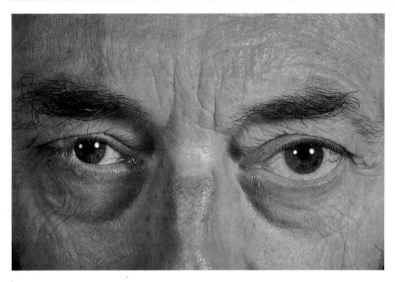

Figure 17.19   Right lateral tarsorrhaphy.

Localized myokymia

The patient experiences a twitching, tic or pulling in the eyelid or in the region of the eye. Only rarely are the contractions pronounced enough to be visible to the observer.

Management   The abnormal movements are usually unexplained and occur in isolation. They are of no serious significance and all that is necessary is to reassure the patient that nothing is wrong.

Spasmodic closure of the lids

The spasmodic closure of the lids may be due to a tic or habit spasm, and occur bilaterally. Hemifacial spasm may include the orbicularis on one side.

Management   Treatment is difficult, but some patients achieve temporary relief from an alcohol injection into the upper branches of the facial nerve at the neck of the mandible, or by infiltration of the orbicularis with botulinum toxin.

PRACTICAL POINTS

● A meibomian cyst if the commonest type of lid swelling. It is usually treated by incision or scraping out of the contents.

● Benign and malignant tumours are not uncommon on the eyelids.

● Secondary staphylococcal infection is common in squamous blepharitis and may lead to styes or infected chalazia.

● Swollen eyelids may indicate an endocrine disorder, general oedema or simply aging.

● Entropion and ectropion of the eyelids are more common in later life. Minor surgical procedures are usually successful in rectifying these problems.

● Ptosis is frequently a hereditary condition and may require cosmetic surgery at an early age.

● Lagophthalmos may lead to exposure of the cornea and protective measures, such as temporary or permanent tarsorrhaphy, may be necessary.

● There is no cure for the occasional spontaneous movements of the eyelids, but these usually occur in episodes that are not prolonged.

18   Eye injuries

It is convenient to discuss eye injuries under three categories:

- Foreign bodies

- Mechanical trauma, either from blunt or from penetrating injuries

- Burns.

Although an eye injury usually falls broadly into one of these groups, it sometimes embraces two of them. For example, a foreign body such as a glass splinter could well cause a penetrating injury of the globe.

FOREIGN BODIES

Foreign bodies commonly give rise to the complaint of 'getting something in the eye'. These usually lodge either on the cornea or under the upper eyelid, the so-called subtarsal foreign body. In both these sites, the foreign body tends to stick and cannot be dislodged by tears or the movement of the lids.

A foreign body on the bulbar conjunctiva does not stick and is usually washed away by the flow of tears, giving rise to nothing more than momentary symptoms which induce blinking and watering, before the foreign body moves on or out of the conjunctival sac.

Corneal foreign body

The presence of a corneal foreign body often occurs industrially, typically after grinding, but may occur in any windy atmosphere (Figure 18.1). The feeling of 'something in the eye' produces blinking and watering, but this may not dislodge the foreign body.

Management   After the eye is anaesthetized with 1 per cent amethocaine drops, the foreign body is picked out. A sharp needle (17 gauge) is used tangentially to the cornea. It should be positioned so as to get behind the foreign body and lever it out. A good light is essential during the procedure, and magnification is helpful.

If the foreign body has been in place for more than a few hours, a ring of brown stain is sometimes evident in the cornea surrounding it. The ring may remain even after the foreign body has been removed. If the eye continues to be irritable, this 'rust ring' (Figure 18.2) may need to be removed separately, a day or two later, by a method similar to that above. In many cases the ring may be left without causing any harm to the eye.

After removal of a corneal foreign body, an antibiotic drop or ointment should be administered. If a great deal of manipulation of the

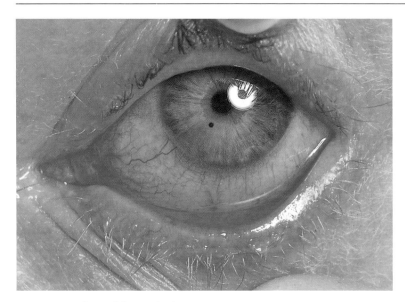

Figure 18.1   Corneal foreign body.

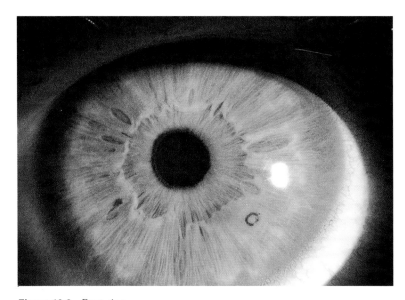

Figure 18.2   Rust ring.

cornea has been necessary, a mydriatic, cyclopentolate (1 per cent), or in more severe cases atropine (1 per cent) should also be instilled. The treatment has the disadvantage of blurring the vision for close work for a variable period of time, even up to a week after atropine is used. This can be a nuisance especially for those very patients whose occupations expose them to risk of corneal foreign bodies.

Whatever medication is used, the eye should be padded and inspected the following day, as occasionally secondary infection may have occurred, producing a localized corneal abscess.

Subtarsal foreign body

A subtarsal foreign body (Figure 18.3) is often produced by wind blowing a particle of dust into the eye.

The dust particle usually settles in the slight concavity of the inner aspect of the upper (the subtarsal groove) 2 mm or so from the edge of the lid. Blinking often fails to dislodge the foreign body and the upper cornea may be irritated as the lid moves.

Management To remove a subtarsal foreign body the upper lid first has to be everted. To carry out the removal of this type of foreign body, the patient looks down and the lashes are held so as to stretch the lid down and forwards. An orange stick or glass rod is then used to press the upper edge of the tarsal plate in the direction of the gap between the lid edge and the globe. By using a rotating manoeuvre, the tarsal plate is everted and the foreign body wiped off. To restore the lid to its normal position, the patient is asked to look upwards (Figure 18.4).

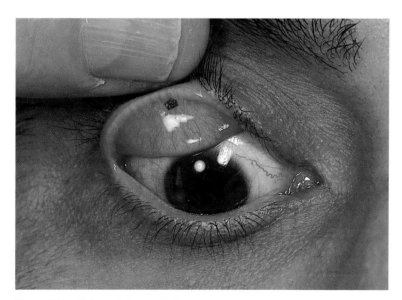

Figure 18.3 Subtarsal foreign body.

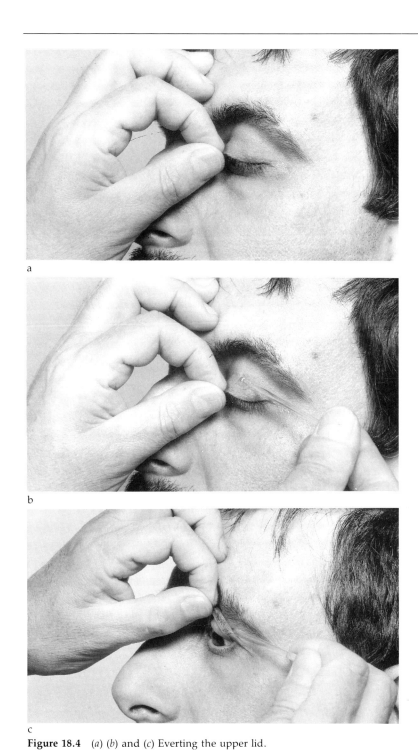

a

b

c

Figure 18.4   (*a*) (*b*) and (*c*) Everting the upper lid.

Intraocular foreign bodies

Intraocular foreign bodies occur rarely but recognition is extremely important. If an intraocular foreign body contains iron and is not removed, the iron will slowly dissolve in the ocular fluid and disseminate throughout the eye, staining the iris brown and destroying the retina and causing glaucoma. The condition is known as siderosis and the eye goes blind.

If a patient presents with 'something in the eye' that is not immediately visible to the physician, it is essential to establish what he or she was doing at the time. If he was hammering or chiselling, the orbit must be x-rayed (Figure 18.5). This is because a tiny metallic fragment can fly off at high speed during this activity and, being hot and probably sterile, can penetrate the coats of the eye, producing only a momentary sensation of a foreign body being present.

The mere suspicion of an intraocular foreign body indicates referral to an ophthalmic surgeon. A specialized examination under high magnification with the slit-lamp is necessary to show where the penetration has occurred. In fact, the patient may remain symptomless for months unless the lens or central retina have been directly involved by the foreign body itself or by its entry track.

Management   Removal of an iron-containing intraocular foreign body is normally carried out with a powerful magnet, or by a direct approach to the part of the eye in which the object has been localized, using x-ray or ultrasound techniques. A full outline of this specialized treatment can be found in the larger texts on ophthalmology (see Bibliography).

For the non-specialist, the most important fact about metallic intraocular foreign bodies is to be always alert to the possibility of their presence, especially in the hammer and chisel type injury.

Obviously operators should be advised to wear protective glasses whenever they are at risk of such an accident. Any case involving an intraocular foreign body may take

infection in with it and chemotherapy is given prophylactically.

BLUNT INJURIES

A blunt injury occurs when the eye or its surrounding structure is struck by an object which does not lodge there but produces a concussion or abrasion of a particular structure.

The following types of injuries may be incurred:

- Lid injuries
- Orbital trauma and fracture
- Injuries to the eyeball itself.

Lid injuries

A common lid injury is a black eye, which is severe bruising of the lids, perhaps with some subconjunctival haemorrhage, often following a direct blow, from a fist, for example (Figure 18.6).

It is frequently difficult to examine the eye properly in these cases because the swelling of the lid is normally severe. If a complete examination is not at first possible, the patient should be seen after a few days when, with the subsiding swelling, the lids can be separated.

Management   No treatment is necessary if there are no other injuries present. The patient may gain psychological comfort from cold compresses.

Laceration of the lids

Laceration of the lids can produce a ghastly-looking injury, but appropriate suturing will frequently produce a satisfactory cosmetic result; attention should be paid to restoring the continuity of the lid margin (Figure 18.7). Particular note must be taken of the inner third of the lids,

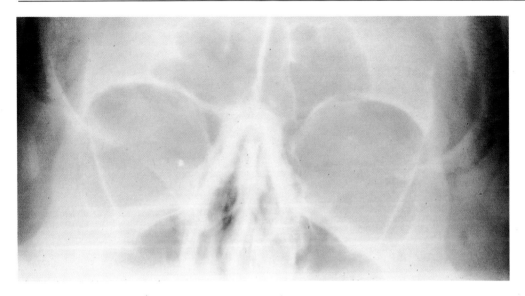

Figure 18.5 An x-ray of the orbits showing an intraocular foreign body on the right side.

especially of the lower lids, because a possible tear in the lacrimal canaliculus may be present. If this is the case, then immediate restoration is necessary. This is not a task for the casualty department of a hospital; rather the services of an ophthalmic surgeon are required because watering of the eye will result as the cut ends of the canaliculus scar.

An x-ray of the facial bones is normally advisable in cases of laceration or severe bruising of the lids. This is because, associated with blunt trauma to the lids, there may be injuries to the orbital bones (see below) and the deformity may be masked by the swollen lids.

Orbital injuries

Orbital fractures may be accompanied by an orbital haemorrhage, as well as direct damage to the orbital structures. The patient may complain of, or show, abnormal protrusion of the eye, or the opposite, and may have diplopia from neuro-muscular involvement. Fractures of the zygoma are common.

An important orbital injury is the 'blow-out' fracture of the orbit as a result of a direct frontal trauma on the globe of the eye (Figure 18.8 and see Figure 16.7). This transmits force to the orbit and cracks the roof of the antrum. Orbital contents may be trapped between the edges of the gap in the bone and, though there are no

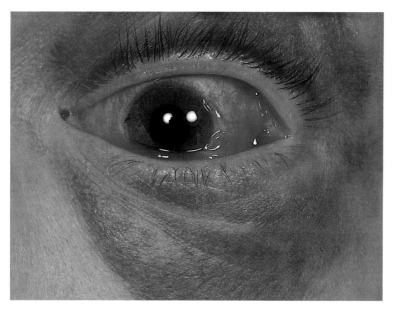

Figure 18.6   A typical black eye–ecchymosis of the lids
and subconjunctival haemorrhage.

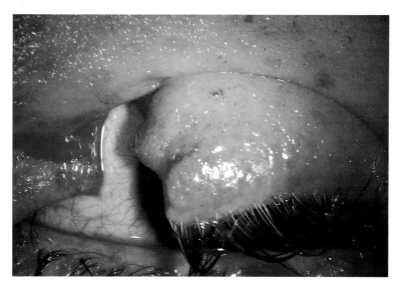

Figure 18.7   A servere lid laceration–the upper lid is
almost completely avulsed and has reversed itself so
that the tarsal plate is facing forwards.

external signs of injury, the eye sinks back and there is restriction of vertical movement, usually of elevation, resulting in diplopia. The infra-orbital nerve may also be damaged, with numbness of the cheek.

Management   Some orbital fractures require the attention of a maxillofacial surgeon. In blow-out fractures, restorative surgery is often best delayed because a surprisingly large element of spontaneous improvement usually occurs.

Surgical approaches vary; one technique is to insert an artificial floor into the orbit, made of silastic sheet, and another is to pad out the antrum, elevating its roof.

Blunt injuries to the eyeball

Blunt injuries may affect any of the eyeball's structures, and are grouped as follows:

- Corneal abrasions
- Hyphaema
- Traumatic iritis
- Traumatic mydriasis

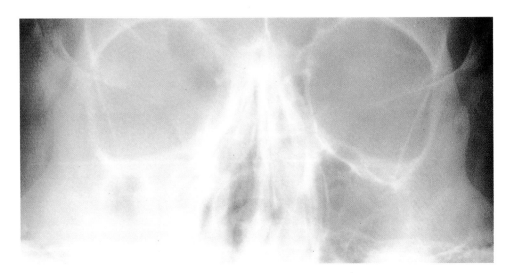

Figure 18.8   An x-ray showing a blow-out fracture of the right orbit. The antrum is opaque and part of the floor and lower orbital contents have prolapsed down into it.

- Lens injuries
- Glaucoma
- Posterior segment injuries
- Massive blunt trauma.

Corneal abrasions

Corneal abrasions (Figure 18.9) are perhaps the commonest non-penetrating injuries to the eyeball, typically produced by infants' fingernails, newsprint, contact lenses, or during gardening (from twigs, etc). The abrasion is very painful, with considerable blepharospasm and watering.

Management   For diagnostic purposes only, a local anaesthetic may be used to examine the eye where fluorescein staining of the area of denuded epithelium is the key sign. If the symptoms are severe, the eye should be padded after administration of antibiotic drops and the mydriatic atropine. In a day or so the epithelium grows over the affected area. The eye should be kept padded until that time.

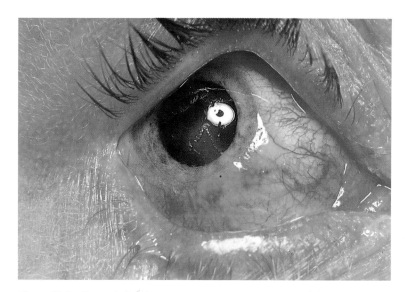

Figure 18.9   Corneal abrasion.

Recurrent corneal abrasion

A recurrent corneal abrasion is sometimes a curious and unpleasant sequel following inadequate healing of an initial injury to the corneal surface. Improperly grounded epithelial cells become detached with the opening of the eyelids typically on waking in the morning. The patient sustains a small abrasion with pain, watering and photophobia and perhaps slight redness. The episode passes off during the course of the day. However, the whole event may be repeated regularly or sporadically, and give rise to considerable anxiety about what is going to happen on opening of the eye after a night's sleep.

Management Lubrication of the eye with methylcellulose drops or 'simple eye ointment',

especially at bedtime, should be carried out for several months, even in the absence of recurrences. Hypertonic sodium chloride 5 per cent, as drops or ointment, has also been suggested. If conservative measures fail, the affected area should be debrided and cauterized with phenol, under local anaesthesia. This procedure is unpleasant for the patient, but usually effects a permanent cure.

Hyphaema

Hyphaema (blood in the anterior chamber) is a frequent result of a modest blunt injury (Figure 18.10). It originates from a minor tear of the iris and may obscure the sight to a considerable degree, at least temporarily. The blood is usually

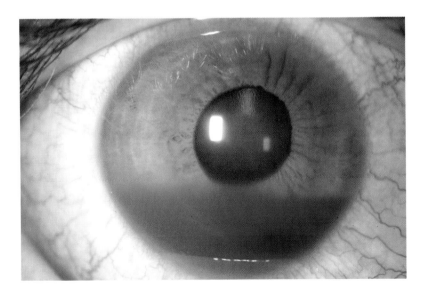

Figure 18.10 A traumatic hyphaema.

absorbed spontaneously, within a few days, but sometimes a secondary haemorrhage occurs. This condition, or even the primary haemorrhage itself, may be accompanied by secondary glaucoma.

Management   Initially the patient should be advised to rest at home. If this is not possible, a short period of hospital bedrest is advisable. Damage to the posterior segment of the eye should be looked for when the clearing of the haemorrhage allows. If there is no evidence of retinal damage, the vision returns to normal once the blood has been completely absorbed.

Traumatic iritis

This condition is an almost universal accompaniment of any significant blunt injury. It may be also associated with some abnormality of the pupil size or reaction. Local steroids are given if the iritis is at all severe. It is usually manifested by the presence of cells and flare in the aqueous humour, visible only by slit-lamp examination.

Traumatic mydriasis

Enlargement of the pupil, sometimes permanent, with poor or absent reactions to light, and accommodation is a frequently encountered sequel to a direct injury to the eye (see Figure 18.6). It is referred to as traumatic mydriasis.

Slight photophobia may be experienced, but the patient's vision may be little affected. No treatment is effective, but some spontaneous recovery is usual.

Lens injuries

A lens injury may result in the lens being displaced or becoming cataractous to some degree (see Chapter 10 and Figure 18.11). Either way, the result is disturbed vision.

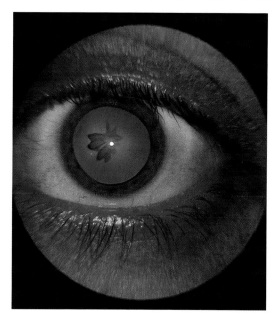

Figure 18.11   A traumatic cataract produced by a blunt injury. The so-called concussion rosette.

Glaucoma

Lens displacement is often accompanied by secondary glaucoma, but the latter is a possible complication of any type of serious blunt injury leading to hyphaema, for example. It can also sometimes be found as an isolated consequence of blunt trauma.

Blunt injury to the posterior segment of the eye

This type of injury often produces a curious oedema of the retina, termed commotio retinae. It can occur anywhere, but particularly affects the macula. If it does happen, then the sight is blurred. The condition usually clears quickly but a degenerative condition or hole may develop which can permanently reduce the vision of the eye.

A choroidoretinal haemorrhage may occur in a severe case of a blunt injury to the eye, and may extend to the vitreous. A retinal tear may result and lead to retinal detachment. This can happen particularly if the retina shows some pre-existing fault as, for example, degenerative changes due to high myopia (see Chapter 7). The management is as for retinal detachment (see Chapter 12).

Massive blunt trauma

Massive blunt trauma may rupture the eyeball. The extensive internal disorganization of the retina leads to blindness in most cases. There is no specific treatment for the condition.

PENETRATING INJURIES

Incised wounds of the globe are always serious. The main cause in civilian life is from an accident involving the shattering of a car windscreen. (Widespread seatbelt legislation appears to have reduced the frequency of these injuries significantly.)

Any incised wound of the globe may be accompanied by prolapse into, or through it, of intraocular contents. Corneal wounds lead to loss of aqueous humour, prolapse of the iris and possible damage to the lens In some cases, this causes immediate cataract formation and tears in the lens capsule, strands of which may attach themselves to the wound, or emerge through it.

Iris prolapse always has a black appearance, whatever the colour of the iris (Figure 18.12). The blackness is due to the colour of the posterior pigmented epithelium, which is the same extremely dark colour in all normal individuals. The pupil is distorted in shape, being elongated towards the prolapse.

Limbal or scleral wounds may be complicated by prolapse of the ciliary body, or of vitreous, occasionally even of choroid or retina.

All penetrating wounds are at risk of secondary infection.

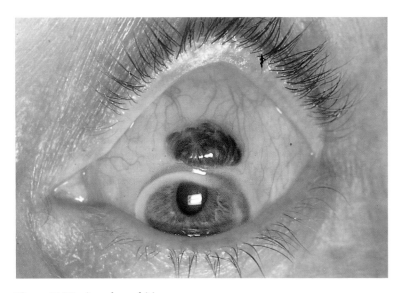

Figure 18.12   A prolapsed iris.

Management   Modern trauma surgery takes the form of a wound toilet and closure by accurate direct edge-to-edge suturing, after removal of as much disturbed intraocular tissue as is appropriate. For example, iris, ciliary body, lens capsule and lens substance (soft lens matter) are all cleared from the wound. In some cases the vitreous may need to be partially or totally removed. Appropriate chemotherapy is given topically and systemically.

A gross penetrating injury will disorganize the globe from the loss of contents and result in collapse of the eyeball, with light perception being negligible or lost. Heroic efforts to restore the eyes are often futile and to preserve them may result only in an unsightly and constantly inflamed organ. This may also bring with it the danger of sympathetic ophthalmia.

Sympathetic ophthalmia

As with blunt injuries, penetration may lead to anterior uveitis. A specific and extremely unpleasant form of uveitis in penetrating injuries may occur first in the injured eye and subsequently in the unaffected fellow eye. This is sympathetic ophthalmia. It usually results from a major incised wound but can also arise in the eye with apparently less serious injuries should these involve the ciliary body, lens capsule and, to a lesser extent, the iris.

Its onset is marked by the development of, or rapid increase in, such symptoms as photophobia, lacrimation and pain in the injured eye, accompanied by similar symptoms in the fellow eye.

Management   Like many forms of uveitis, sympathetic ophthalmia is responsive to steroids, though far less so than the usual type of uveitis. When rampant, it involves all the uvea in both eyes, leading to bilateral blindness. This is best avoided by a prudent and timely decision being made on whether to preserve a badly injured eye. Such a decision is often difficult and depends on an assessment of the degree of

vision likely to be obtained from the eye, when it recovers, as against the danger of leaving it in situ.

BURNS

Thermal burns

Thermal burns may be of any severity, from a slight charring of the eyelashes to a horrific destruction of the eyelids with direct involvement of the globe, particularly the cornea, or with indirect effects on the globe owing to the failure of the lids to close.

Management   In the latter cases, the cornea must be kept moist. For this a soft contact lens may be helpful. Where scarring of the lids leads to lagophthalmos, plastic reconstruction is necessary. In milder cases, local steroids, antibiotics and mydriatics are applied copiously to the eye and the lids.

Chemical burns

These burns may scar the lids, cornea or conjunctiva, or all of them.

A sealing together of the raw conjunctival surfaces of the globe and lid (symblepharon) may partly or wholly immobilize the eyeball. Conjunctival scarring may also seal off the lacrimal gland, leading to dryness, which aggravates an already existing conjunctival and corneal problem.

The immediate effect of the chemical on the cornea is to cause ulceration and there may be penetration of the substance into the anterior chamber, causing iritis or cataract. The chemically inflamed cornea may become vascularized in time and finally scarred with consequent loss of vision.

A particular chemical burn which often produces injuries in the building trade is lime, which has an unpleasant habit of adhering in particles to the conjunctival surface (Figure 18.13). Such

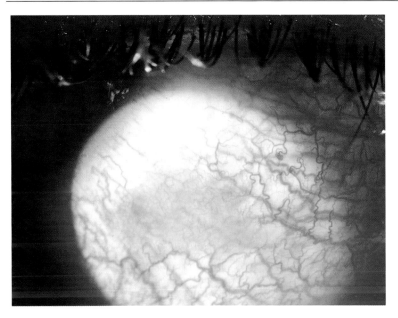

Figure 18.13 An area of chemical abrasion of the conjunctiva due to lime; stained with fluorescein. Note that loss of conjunctival surface stains yellow as against the green colour of corneal epithelial loss.

injuries appear trivial when first seen, but patients should have expert inspection since serious effects may be delayed. Close inspection may reveal not only fragments of lime that are difficult to remove, but also widespread chemical destruction of the epithelium of the conjunctiva and cornea.

Management In dealing with such burns in an emergency, no attempt should be made to search for a specific antidote. Instead there should be copious irrigation with water or saline. After this, local antibiotics and steroids, and mydriatics are instilled. Separation of the raw conjunctival surface is maintained with a glass rod or by insertion of a contact lens. Ascorbic acid given topically and systemically is said to be helpful.

After the acute phase is over, an assessment is made of the effects of any scarring of the lids, the cornea or the conjunctiva. If corneal scarring leads to significant loss of vision, which cannot be improved by spectacles or contact lenses, corneal grafting may be needed.

Physical injury

This type of eye injury may occur as a result of excessive exposure to light waves other than those in the visible spectrum. If the patient has been exposed to ultraviolet light, this may lead to one of two conditions:

● Eczematous reaction of the eyelids, the equivalent to a vigorous form of sunburn

● Excessive exposure to ultraviolet light, as in arc welding (arc eye), unprotected use of sunlamps, or in skiing (so-called 'snow blindness') may, in some circumstances, affect the eye itself.

A typical result is an acute oedema of the corneal epithelium, which produces an intensely photophobic and painful eye. Both eyes are usually affected.

Management   Eczema of the lids may be treated by antihistamine or steroid ointment. Acute oedema of the corneal epithelium is best avoided by wearing suitable protective glasses or shields. Once the condition has occurred, it is simply treated with a short-term mydriatic and padding of both eyes. The corneal epithelium will restore itself to normal within twenty-four hours.

Prevention of all types of eye injury is through wearing suitable protection in the form of goggles, shatterproof spectacles and glasses of an appropriate tint. Avoiding hazardous occupations and activities wherever possible, and the wearing of seatbelts by car passengers in rear as well as front seats are strongly advised.

PRACTICAL POINTS

● Externally lodging foreign bodies are either on the cornea or under the upper lid.

● Intraocular foreign bodies are rare, but particular attention should be paid to a history of hammering and chiselling.

● Corneal abrasion is a common and extremely painful condition. It is best to pad up the eye, having given some drops to dilate the pupil, as well as an antibiotic.

● Severe blunt injuries may be marked by bleeding into the lids, into the conjunctiva or into the anterior chamber—a hyphaema. The view of the back of the eye may be difficult in the early stages of the management of such cases, but there may be injury to the retina as well as to the lens, producing a traumatic cataract.

● Penetrating injuries of the anterior segment of the eye will often be marked by an irregularity of the pupil and perhaps a loss of the anterior chamber as the aqueous humour escapes.

● Surgery of such cases requires the debridement of the wound, removing any incarcerated iris, ciliary body, lens matter or vitreous. The wound itself is then sutured under microscopy.

● Chemical injuries should be treated by copious irrigation in the emergency situation. A particularly important industrial injury is produced by lime. All such patients should be referred for hospital management.

19 Strabismus, lazy eyes and double vision

Strabismus is a condition where the two eyes do not look at the same object. The deviation in direction of gaze of the two eyes is most commonly in the horizontal plane, usually convergent – esotropia – the two eyes being turned towards each other, and if one eye is persistently deviating it appears to be turned in towards the nose. In the less frequent cases of divergent squints – exotropia – the eyes are turned away from each other and one eye looks as if it is turned outwards. Vertical deviations – hypertropia – are comparatively rare. Whatever the direction of the strabismus, it is important to differentiate between those that arise in childhood and those that originate in later life.

Concomitant or paralytic strabismus?

Childhood strabismus

A strabismus discovered in childhood is usually of the **concomitant** ('moving together') type: the disparity in the line of view of the two eyes remains constant in whichever direction they turn. There is no associated paralysis of movement in any particular direction of either eye. The eye muscles are healthy, but respond to inappropriate innervational stimuli.

Adult strabismus

In later life (and uncommonly in childhood) a strabismus of a **paralytic** or incomitant type may develop. The movement, usually of one eye, in a particular direction is restricted. When the individual looks in that direction a very marked strabismus is present. Looking in the opposite direction, the eyes are straight. Thus, in paralytic strabismus the angle of the deviation will vary according to the direction of the gaze.

Most adults with strabismus have the concomitant type which arose during childhood and has been present ever since.

Consequences of strabismus

The consequences of strabismus depend on the degree of the development of binocular vision at the time of the onset. In simple terms, binocular vision is the transmission of neural impulses from the two eyes to the brain, representing similar images from the retinae, and the entry of a fused single picture into consciousness. To maintain the picture as single, the central nervous system instructs the ocular musculature to maintain the position of the eyes so that the images are similar enough to be fused into one.

Three elements are therefore essential for normal binocular vision:

1 Individual clear images from the two eyes

2 The central nervous fusion mechanism

3 The efferent motor apparatus.

The complex is partly inborn and reinforced by use in early life. If anything prevents this early reinforcement, or the binocular vision is disrupted, the system may never become fully functional or may be completely abandoned.

If the two eyes look in different directions in early life, making the images presented to the brain so dissimilar that the process of fusion is impossible, then the image from one eye is suppressed to avoid confusion. This is how an amblyopic or 'lazy eye' can originate, arising in early life when the binocular vision is incompletely developed. Amblyopia is therefore likely in a case of strabismus developing before the age of five years. It affects only the deviating eye and it is important to remember that the vision of the eye is poor, even when a clear image is focused on its quite normal retina.

In the adult, whose binocular process is fully functional, taking notice of both images is mandatory; so when a strabismus producing two different images develops, diplopia (double vision) results. Neither image can be suppressed in consciousness.

Amblyopia and diplopia are thus counterparts and whether one or the other is a consequence of strabismus depends on how developed the binocular powers are, this in turn depending on the age at which the squint starts.

It should be appreciated that a child's strabismus often presents as a cosmetic complaint, any visual defect being unnoticed and double vision not experienced; in the adult with a strabismus that has not been present since childhood, double vision is the main symptom.

Common varieties of strabismus

The two commonest presentations of childhood and adult types are:

• Concomitant convergent strabismus, occurring in early childhood

• VIth nerve malfunction, commonly arising in adult life and leading to paralytic strabismus.

Concomitant convergent strabismus

This type of childhood strabismus (Figure 19.1) occurs between two and four years of age, against the optical background of hypermetropia (see Chapter 7).

The association with long-sightedness stems from the relationship between the accommodation, focusing on a near object, which hypermetropes use to excess to give clear retinal images, and convergence, used to turn the eye towards a nearer object; both functions are necessary for clear, near viewing.

The degree of accommodation and convergence are roughly related. This relationship is disturbed if accommodation is already being used for distance vision.

The hypermetrope's excessive accommodation tends to drive up the convergence. The tendency to turn the eye inwards is resisted by the power of the binocular vision, which holds the images similar. If binocular vision is incompletely developed, it may not be sustainable and a convergent strabismus results.

VIth (abducens) nerve malfunction

This type of strabismus arises in later adult life, and causes double vision with the two images separated horizontally. It is often sudden in onset. The nerve malfunction producing the condition is described in Chapter 23.

There can be many neurological causes, but in most cases no systemic cause is found.

Examination

Apart from a general examination, three special procedures should be carried out during an examination for strabismus:

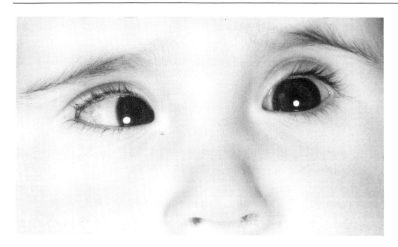

Figure 19.1 Right convergent squint. Notice the outward displacement of the right corneal reflection.

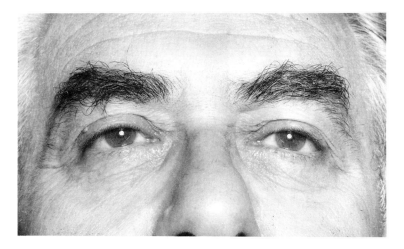

Figure 19.2 Normal eyes with central corneal reflections.

1 **Inspection of the corneal reflections** The examiner asks the patient to look at a small light source and notes the position of the reflection of this light from the cornea (Figure 19.2). The reflection is normally either central in relation to the pupil, or symmetrically eccentric from the two eyes.

If the reflection is eccentric, or much more eccentric from one eye, then this suggests that a strabismus is present.

2 **A simple cover test** If it is suspected that one eye is deviating, the patient is again asked to look at ('fix') a particular object. The

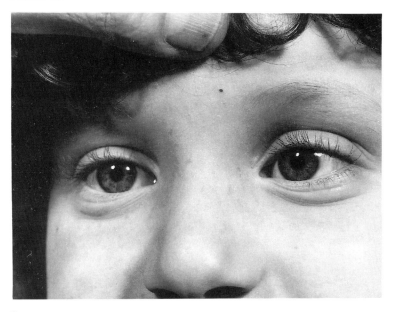

a

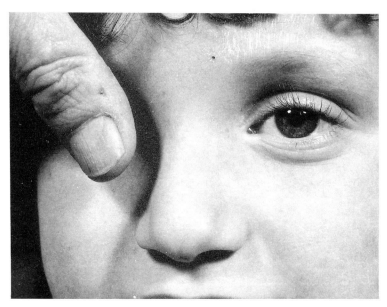

b

Figure 19.3 The cover test: (*a*) shows a left convergent
squint; (*b*) shows that on covering the right eye the left
eye has to move outwards to take up fixation,
indicating its originally convergent position.

non-deviating eye is then covered by the hand or a card (Figure 19.3). The suspected eye will be seen to move to take up fixation if a true strabismus is present. More complex versions of the cover test can be performed, for example, the cover is passed from eye to eye and what happens to each eye under cover is observed. This may reveal a latent strabismus (see page 192).

3 **Examination of the ocular movements** (Figure 19.4) The patient is asked to follow an object while keeping the head still. The ability to move the eyes in any of nine directions is noted, and the patient is asked whether the object becomes double in any particular direction. The nine directions are: straight ahead, right and left, then up centre, right and left and finally down centre, right and left.

The first two procedures suggest whether a true strabismus is present. The third indicates whether it is concomitant or paralytic. If the strabismus is paralytic, examination of the eye movements will show the direction in which the strabismus is most marked. It also reveals where the doubled images are most widely separated, which is always in the direction of action of the paralysed muscle or muscles.

The general eye examination carried out on an adult will follow the customary routine of vision assessment, as well as inspection of the anterior and posterior segments of the eye. In a child, these examinations may not be entirely possible—often owing to lack of cooperation—without special methods for assessing vision (see Chapter 25) and inspecting the eye itself.

Important features of concomitant strabismus

There are a number of important features to be noted in concomitant strabismus:

1 A family history is often present (Figure 19.5).

2 Children do not grow out of strabismus. What they do grow out of is the false appearance of the condition (pseudostrabismus) produced by a flat nose bridge or by epicanthic folds, or both (Figure 19.6). The condition is very often mistakenly believed by patients or relatives to be a convergent strabismus.

3 Amblyopia, predominantly a feature of unilateral convergent strabismus, can be treated by covering (occlusion) the straight eye, thereby forcing attention on the image from the deviating eye. This is most successful if done within a reasonably short time of onset. Early referral is essential and parents should never be told that the child is too young for treatment or will grow out of the condition. Even babies under one year of age can be occluded and given spectacles, or operated upon. Amblyopia is largely avoidable by early diagnosis and treatment. Failure to recognize the condition leads to an unhappy situation in later life if the unaffected eye becomes injured or diseased.

4 The degree of strabismus is irrelevant in the development of amblyopia. A small degree of convergence may be cosmetically acceptable, but this is just as likely to cause amblyopia as a deviation of a larger degree.

5 Strabismus may be truly congenital. A special variety of congenital concomitant strabismus is the alternating type in which one eye may fix, and the switch over to the other occurs spontaneously and frequently. As each eye is at some time in use, the other being temporarily suppressed, the individual vision when tested is found to be good on both sides. Amblyopia does not occur in either eye and occlusion is not needed. In some of these cases there is a history of obstetric difficulty.

6 It is important to be aware that strabismus in a child may indicate that the eye is functionally poor from an organic disease (such as congenital cataract or retinal anomaly). Remember, therefore, that an eye

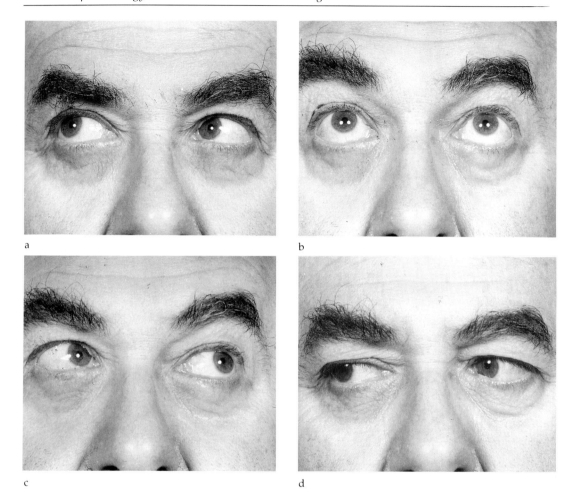

a

b

c

d

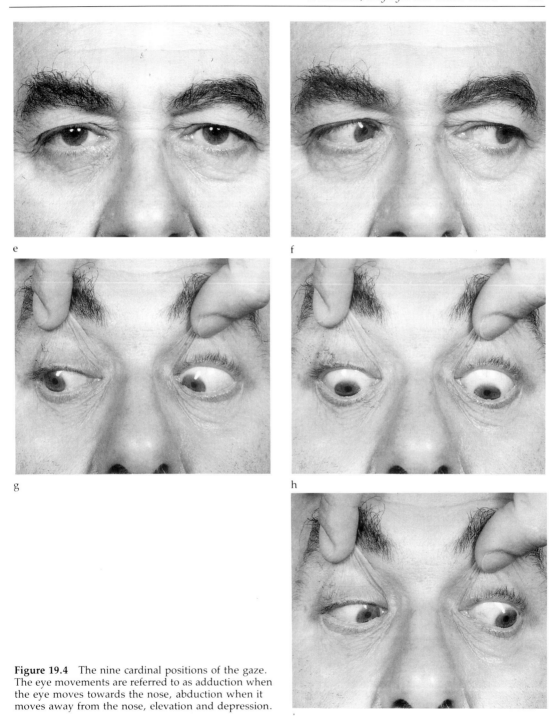

Figure 19.4 The nine cardinal positions of the gaze. The eye movements are referred to as adduction when the eye moves towards the nose, abduction when it moves away from the nose, elevation and depression.

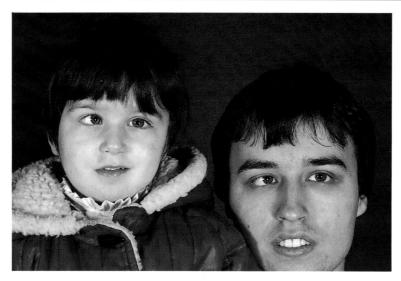

Figure 19.5 Concomitant strabismus is often familial. A father and daughter, both with right concomitant convergent strabismus.

with strabismus may not see well owing to amblyopia, but also that an eye which does not see well owing to an organic disease may develop a strabismus.

Management of concomitant strabismus

This applies particularly to the common convergent type and to the rather less frequent divergent variety.

After it has been established that a true strabismus is present, a simple examination of the eyes is necessary to ensure they are organically healthy. The pupil reactions should be noted and an examination made of the retina and optical state of the patient. This is normally undertaken after a cycloplegic (accommodation-paralysing) drug has been administered (for example, atropine 1 per cent drops or ointment), often for a few days before examination.

If found necessary at the examination, spectacles are prescribed, to be worn full time. The patient should then be investigated by an orthoptist, who will measure the direction and degree of the strabismus, assess the individual vision of the two eyes, and attempt to discover whether any binocular cooperation is possible. A synoptophore, an instrument which presents different images to the two eyes, is used (Figure 19.7). If the images can be combined to any

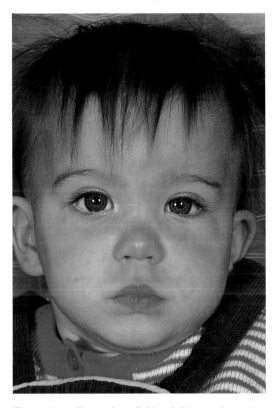

Figure 19.6 Epicanthus. Folds of skin run from the upper to the lower lid, covering the medial aspect of the white of the eye and giving a false impression of left convergence.

degree, some binocular power exists. This power is graded into three levels:

1 Simultaneous perception, which is a basic ability to see two sets of images at the same time, rather than alternately

2 The power to fuse the images

3 Stereoscopic perception (three-dimensional) of the fused images.

If one eye is discovered to be amblyopic, which is usually the case if the strabismus is persistently present in one eye, the fixing eye is occluded (Figure 19.8). Occlusion is not necessary if the strabismus is of the uncommon alternating type (see above). Such cases may proceed directly to surgery for cosmetic reasons.

Over the succeeding weeks and months, the follow-up may show improvement in the vision of the deviating eye, through the help of spectacles and occlusion.

Once vision has improved maximally, surgery may be indicated to improve the appearance, or to restore binocular vision if there is a reasonable chance of this.

Much of the preoperative supervision is by an orthoptist who, as well as monitoring the effect of occlusion in improving the vision, may also give exercises 'on the synoptophore' to improve binocular powers. These exercises are not to strengthen a weak muscle; indeed this is simply not possible, as muscle weakness is not part of the existing condition of concomitant strabismus. Such an intention is as misguided as that for various other forms of eye exercise suggested, for example, to alleviate myopia.

In summary, the ophthalmologist and orthoptist have three objectives in the treatment of concomitant strabismus. The first is the improvement of vision of each eye individually. The second is to establish or restore the power of binocular vision, and the third to attend to the cosmetic aspect.

The second aim is the hardest to achieve, dependent as it is, at least partially, on attaining the first. In other words, getting good binocular vision can only result from good individual vision, and occlusion to improve the sight of an amblyopic eye may turn out to be only partially effective.

Finally, a word of caution on the results of surgery. When this is undertaken for cosmetic reasons only, the patient should be warned that

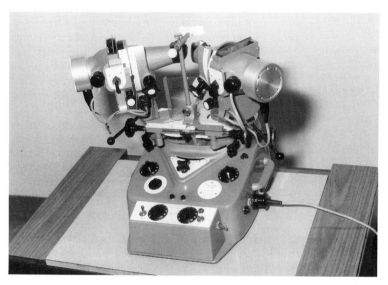

Figure 19.7 The synoptophore.

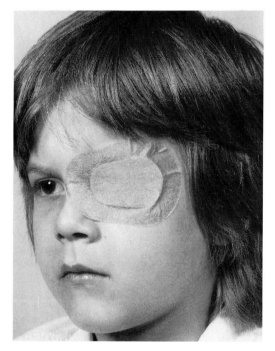

Figure 19.8 Occlusion of a child with a right convergent squint. The left eye is covered in order to force the right eye into use.

the vision of an irretrievably amblyopic eye will not be improved. This applies particularly to adults undergoing cosmetic surgery for a concomitant strabismus that arose in childhood.

Important features of paralytic strabismus

The actions of the eye muscles and their investigation are important in paralytic strabismus. The complaint of double vision is investigated to determine which of the six extrinsic ocular muscles is affected (Figure 19.9). As many of these cases are neurological in origin, a simple clinical examination technique is given in Part 3 (see Chapter 23). Further investigation is always carried out by an orthoptist, so only the principles are outlined below:

● The two images will be farthest apart in the direction of the action of the paralysed muscle

• The farthest displaced image is from the eye with the muscle weakness

• Double vision can be charted and its extent reassessed at intervals.

The interpretation of double vision is simple in respect of the horizontally acting muscles. The medial rectus normally turns the eye nasally and the lateral rectus turns the eye outwards. When either of these is defective, the images from the two eyes are horizontally separated.

When the vertically acting muscles are involved, the diplopia takes the form of vertically or diagonally separated images, making interpretation more difficult. This is due to the complex actions of the vertically acting muscles. A straight, upward movement of the eyes is produced principally by the superior rectus, some of its ancillary actions (rotation and adduction) being cancelled out by a simultaneous action of the inferior oblique. A synergy of the inferior rectus and superior oblique muscles produces the converse, downward movement. In combined horizontal and vertical movement, the appropriate rectus or oblique muscles will predominate. This allows a differential diagnosis by analysis of diplopia occurring in the diagonal movements of the eye. Typically, a right IVth (trochlear) nerve palsy would cause weakness of the right superior oblique muscle, producing diplopia with the images vertically separated and maximally when looking down and to the left; this is because the depressor action of the right superior oblique is greater on left gaze.

As might be expected, the pattern of diplopia becomes even more complicated when there is a weakness of more than one muscle, particularly a combination of horizontally and vertically acting muscles.

Management of paralytic strabismus

A full general medical, cardiovascular and neurological investigation is necessary in a case of a

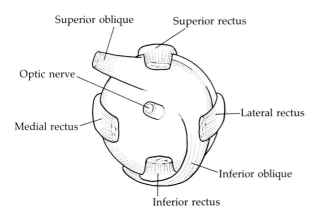

Figure 19.9 A diagrammatic representation of the eye muscles and their attachments to the eyeball. This is a rear view of the right eyeball.

paralytic strabismus. This is because the strabismus may be primarily neurogenic or myogenic (a result of dysthyroid disease or myasthenia gravis, for example).

In the commonest type of paralytic strabismus, which is a sudden lateral rectus weakness causing poor outward movement, spontaneous recovery can be expected within two to three months. Occlusion is indicated in any case of diplopia, at least as a temporary measure to avoid confusion. It is best to cover the eye or blank out the spectacle lens on the side with the muscle weakness.

Persistent paralysis, from whatever cause, may justify prismatic spectacles, even if an orthoptic examination reveals the degree of paralysis to be unstable. Such prisms may be stuck on to the patient's own glasses.

Surgery may be advised if diplopia cannot be adequately reduced by prisms and restoration to a binocular state is thought possible. It may not be feasible to restore a full binocular field, but the aim should be to abolish diplopia in the straight ahead and downward directions of the gaze.

Surgery for strabismus

The principles of surgery for strabismus, whether concomitant or paralytic, are similar. The muscle acting in the direction of the deviation is weakened by moving backwards its insertion on the eyeball; this is known as recession. The antagonist of this muscle is strengthened by effectively advancing its insertion (Figure 19.10). It may be necessary to combine this with the removal of a small portion of the tendon, the procedure known as resection.

In a typical operation for concomitant convergent strabismus of 20 degrees, the medial rectus insertion would be recessed 5 mm and the lateral rectus resected 6 to 7 mm.

Intermittent and latent strabismus

One type of inconstant strabismus (see page 190) is paralytic strabismus where the degree of disparity of the lines of view of the two eyes vary with the direction of the gaze. Even concomitant strabismus may be inconstant in time. The onset of many cases of concomitant strabismus in childhood is often gradual, the deviation being present only when the child is tired. At other times, the binocular powers that have already developed will pull the eyes straight. The mere history of a strabismus is therefore a sufficient enough reason for referral.

The intermittent feature of concomitant strabismus may persist into adult life. Instead of the deviation becoming manifest permanently, or for any length of time, a tenuous binocularity is always present, the strabismus being latent. There may be a tendency for the eye to deviate and, with adult quality binocular vision, this may lead to temporary diplopia. It is also possible for this tendency to give rise to the symptoms of eyestrain (see Chapter 4).

Nevertheless, although mild cases of latent strabismus are widespread, they are often symptomless. The discovery of the condition, in the absence of any complaint, is not an indication to take any particular course of action. In patients who do have symptoms that might be related to a latent muscle imbalance, it is often difficult to decide whether these symptoms (often vague in nature) are really due to the muscle problem. Clinical judgement is needed to decide the relevance of the objective findings.

The varieties of latent strabismus parallel the manifest varieties. Hence the terms for the conditions are: latent strabismus—esophoria; latent divergence—exophoria; and latent vertical deviation—hyperphoria. These conditions are revealed by a modification of the cover test. Initially both eyes are looking at the fixing light. When one is covered, that eye deviates while the other remains fixed; on uncovering, the deviated eye returns to fixation. The same usually happens when the covering and uncovering is carried out on the other eye. The condition is thus symmetrical.

The assessment of latent strabismus is often accompanied by the optical investigation of the patient (refraction) by an optician or ophthalmologist. Special devices are used to measure the degree of latent strabismus.

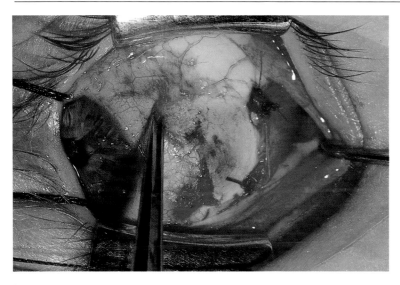

a

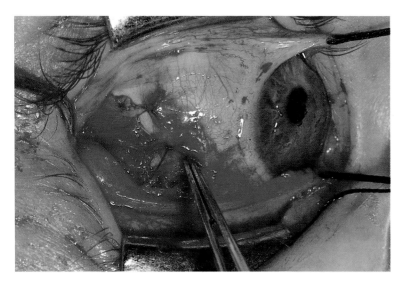

b

Figure 19.10 Strabismus surgery: (*a*) shows the recession of the right medial rectus. The original and final insertions of the muscle are separated by a grey area of sclera. (*b*) shows a resection where the lateral rectus is pulled forward to make its action more advantageous.

The further investigation of these cases proceeds as for manifest strabismus.

Common varieties of intermittent strabismus

Latent divergence and convergence weakness
Latent divergence for near vision is sometimes associated with weakness of convergence. While the conditions may exist independently, both can give rise to difficulty with reading and it is in this particular incoordination that orthoptic eye exercises claim their greatest success.

The patient is taught to fix on an object such as a pencil held in his hand and then slowly bring it towards the eye until he sees a double image. Normally, convergence without diplopia is possible to a distance of about 10 cm from the eye. In convergence weakness, double vision will occur much farther away. As soon as it occurs, the object should be moved out until it becomes single, and then brought forward again.

By repeating this procedure, the near point of convergence gradually approaches closer to the normal position. Similar exercises can be given more formally on the synoptophore.

The value of eye exercises for conditions other than strabismus (to abolish the need for spectacles for refractive errors, for example) is not an accepted procedure in orthodox ophthalmology.

In all cases of intermittent strabismus, significant refractive errors are corrected by spectacles; latent divergence is often accompanied by myopia, for example. Some cases of latent strabismus may be helped by prisms being incorporated in the correction. If this form of treatment is unacceptable or unhelpful to the patient, surgery may have to be considered.

Accommodative strabismus A particular variety of intermittent strabismus which should be noted is a type due to over-accommodation. In this form, which also occurs in children, the eyes are straight on distant gaze, but one eye turns in markedly on close viewing.

To reduce this faulty accommodation, bifocal spectacles or pilocarpine eyedrops (given to reduce the need to exert accommodation) may be tried. Surgery has some advocates, but it may correct the deviation for near vision by producing a deviation for distance. Fortunately, with time, there is a tendency for the problem to become less marked.

PRACTICAL POINTS

● There are two principal types of strabismus, concomitant, where the eyes move together and the angle of squint remains the same whatever the direction of gaze, and paralytic in which the angle of squint varies according to the direction of gaze, and is most marked in the direction of action of the paralysed muscle.

● Concomitant squint arises only in childhood. The squinting eye may become amblyopic, its image being suppressed in order to avoid double vision.

● Early referral of all cases of strabismus is advisable. Preoperative management is by an orthoptist.

● Children do not grow out of a true squint.

● The angle of strabismus is not relevant to the development of amblyopia. Any eye that is not coordinated with its fellow may become amblyopic if the strabismus develops early enough in life.

● The characteristic symptom of paralytic strabismus developing in an adult who has already attained full binocular vision, is the complaint of double vision.

● Paralytic strabismus may have important neurological associations, whereas concomitant strabismus is a condition of its own and has no necessary general association.

● In childhood, the treatment for amblyopia is occlusion. This is not likely to be successful after the age of seven or eight years, but much depends on how longstanding the condition is.

● Surgery to straighten a strabismus may be undertaken at any age, but if one eye is amblyopic, straightening by surgery will not improve the vision of that eye.

● It is important to remember that very occasionally a strabismus presents in a child as the first sign of organic disease of the deviating eye.

● Latent strabismus and convergence weakness may cause eye strain.

PART 3: INTERRELATIONSHIPS OF OPHTHALMOLOGY

Following the clinical orientation of Part 2, the first chapter in Part 3 discusses continuing care, with particular reference to specialization and prophylaxis. The important subject of drug therapy in relation to ophthalmology is reviewed in the second chapter.

Subsequent chapters are concerned with the interaction between ophthalmology and other disciplines, especially the major ones of general medicine and neurology.

20   Continuing management and prophylaxis

Continuing management in ophthalmology includes:

- Routine checks of the eyes and vision
- Management of non-optical cases
- Specialist care
- Social services.

Routine checks of the eyes and vision

The majority of eye cases are simple refractive errors that normally come under the care of the opticians, and usually remain under their care without the need for medical intervention, unless any other condition develops. So do such cases require regular check-ups?

If the patient has serviceable spectacles which provide him with adequate distance and near vision, and he is in good general health with no family history of serious eye disease, then check-ups are not necessary. The idea of a regular two or three yearly check-up throughout life is simply not tenable. However, there are periods in life when a regular examination is indicated:

1 All newly born infants should have a routine inspection of the eyes.

2 Pre-school children should be observed in 'baby clinics' for obvious visual difficulty and for strabismus as part of a routine general assessment.

3 Early in schooling all children should have an eye examination to establish the standard of vision and to identify any refractive errors, or any lazy eye or strabismus problems. Spectacles are given, if needed.

4 An ophthalmologist should see all children at least once to ensure there are no serious organic diseases present; subsequent supervision by opticians is perfectly satisfactory if no organic disease is revealed. Definite strabismus or other organic disease, and some very high refractive errors, should be managed only by an ophthalmologist.

5 Routine re-examination of schoolchildren is important because of the possible development of myopia around the age of ten years. Myopia normally increases in degree during adolescence, and so re-examination of all myopes at intervals of, say, two school terms is most important.

6 Routine checks of adults who have no visual complaints are not necessary between the

ages of twenty and forty years. The subsequent development and increase of presbyopia may require a two to three yearly check-up, but it is often better simply to leave it to the patient to come for a further assessment as and when the reading difficulty is re-experienced even when the current spectacles are used.

7 At a later stage, for adults, there is again no reason for dogged re-attendance unless there is a need for reassessment; for example, if there is a family history of glaucoma or cataract in later life. The fact that some opticians are equipped to perform routine tonometry should not necessarily be regarded as a reason for all middle-aged patients to attend for re-examination unless there is good reason to do so.

8 In the elderly, there is perhaps a case for routine screening by social service personnel, if not by opticians or ophthalmologists. Many elderly people are housebound or confined to homes for the elderly, and slow deterioration of vision may go unrecognized. Screening sometimes leads to the discovery of a treatable cataract, or glaucoma.

Management of non-optical cases

Management of non-optical cases falls into several categories:

1 Cases that require continuous supervision by an ophthalmologist; for example, cases of primary glaucoma and some intractable or recurrent inflammatory conditions of the eye

2 Those cases requiring a short period of intensive management following surgery for cataract or retinal detachment, for example

3 Mild conditions of the outer eye, as, for example, simple bacterial conjunctivitis, that can soon be discharged altogether.

Few cases of any significant clinical condition are returned to the general physician for continued care. They are managed by the staff of the eye department in a general hospital, or a special eye hospital. This is partly because the specialized apparatus and examination techniques needed are simply not available in general practice.

Specialist care: eye departments and eye hospitals

The eye department of a general hospital is usually a minor model of an eye hospital proper. It is likely to have more routine work and less in the way of specialized techniques of diagnosis and investigation, unless one or more of its medical staff has a particular interest. The members of an eye department will, however, inevitably see many more of the ophthalmic associations of general disease than the specialist hospital.

In one respect, the eye department and the eye hospital are similar. The bulk of in-patient work is likely to be of a surgical nature, while most non-surgical ophthalmology is managed on an out-patient basis.

Ophthalmic surgery

As discussed in Part 1, this is the province of the ophthalmic surgeon alone. The most obvious distinction between ophthalmic surgery and other branches of surgery is its small scale. Corresponding to this, the specialized instruments needed call for very high standards of manufacture and durability, as well as ease of manipulation of both tissue and suture material.

Cutting instruments make use of disposable blades or of 'permanent' material, as in diamond knives. Forceps need expert hand finishing to ensure alignment of blades and teeth. Delicacy of handling by the surgeon and theatre staff ensures minimum insult to the ocular tissues and a longer working life for the instruments themselves.

Microscopy is now almost universal in any procedure involving the anterior segment of the eyeball as, for example, in cataract, glaucoma and corneal surgery; it is essential in the new operations on the vitreous, or on the retina from within the globe.

Microscopy is also mandatory when there is a need to handle very fine suture materials and needles, many of which are almost invisible to the naked eye. Indeed, the closure of wounds involving incision of the structural coats of the eye (the cornea and sclera) has been so far improved by microsurgical techniques that there has been a revolution in postoperative care.

Bedrest is hardly necessary and the length of stay in hospital is being progressively reduced, and for some procedures abolished. Corresponding to this, the need for specialized ophthalmic nursing skills has become more theatre and much less ward orientated.

In the theatre, the usual skills in handling delicate instruments have been increasingly amplified by familiarity with the complex and often changing apparatus and surgical methods. In cataract surgery, for instance, a modern ophthalmic nurse needs to be acquainted with the apparatus for cryotherapy, phaco-emulsification, irrigation and aspiration of the anterior chamber, as well as numerous types of intraocular lens.

In vitreous and detachment surgery, more specialized techniques are being added to the standard complex of silicone 'stitch-ons' and bands. Equally, the approach to the retina from within promises yet more elaborate methods involving the use of highly individual instruments and techniques for operative examination and treatment.

Superspecialization

There is an increasing trend towards a narrowing of interests of many ophthalmologists. Certainly in major centres, particularly in the USA, super-specialization is now the norm and there are experts in particular facets of ophthalmology (in glaucoma or retinal disease, for example). In the USA, it is now common practice to become an expert in one branch of ophthalmology to the

virtual exclusion of all others. The pros and cons of such an arrangement are beyond the scope of this book.

Social services

Severe, irretrievable and progressive loss of vision may eventually take a patient beyond the care of the ophthalmologist. At this stage, as well as before, the social services (both statutory and voluntary) play an enormous and important role in the adjustment and rehabilitation of the blind and partially sighted.

In all developed countries, numerous organizations exist to make available all the appropriate advice and facilities.

In the home, advice on lighting and visual aids is given for those who are partially sighted; for example, large dial telephones, talking books and entertainment by radio, these days often with special programmes for their partial disability, as well as by tapes, can be provided.

In more severe loss of vision, the Braille or Moon embossed tactile types may be learned for reading, as well as the use of more sophisticated methods such as the optical tactile converter (a camera which changes print into a palpable pattern) and, most recently, an electronic camera that reads print aloud using a synthetic voice. Outdoors, the provision of a white stick and, where advisable, a guide dog, is arranged.

Blindness in the younger age groups calls for counselling on suitable training and employment. This is now often undertaken on a residential basis.

Statutory registration for both the blind and the partially sighted is an essential preliminary to such training. It is also important in the older age groups to ensure that the relevant authorities are aware of the visually handicapped in their area of care.

Prophylaxis

A realistic view of preventive ophthalmology must emphasize its limitations. Admittedly there are important eye diseases caused by eradicable or avoidable infections, but otherwise many of the major conditions such as senile cataract and macular degeneration are poorly understood as to their aetiology and at present offer no scope for prophylaxis.

There are some exceptions, of course, and these have been noted in sections of Part 2. Routine tonometry is very important in the detection and prevention of chronic simple glaucoma. Examination and treatment of the fellow eye is vital in cases of closed angle glaucoma, and also of retinal detachment. Some of the serious inherited retinal disorders may be prevented by genetic counselling.

Other suggested prophylactic measures are less well established. Is excessive reading to be avoided in the developing myope? Should all children have routine refraction early in life in order to prevent amblyopia? What is the relationship of excellent diabetic control, justifiable of course in itself, to the development or rather the hoped for absence of retinopathy? There are no categorical answers to these questions. In the case of ocular trauma, the place of sensible precautions, such as protective goggles or simple avoidance of dangerous activities, is unquestioned.

PRACTICAL POINTS

● Routine checks of visual acuity are necessary only in early life and for the very elderly, among whom defects may go unnoticed.

● Management of chronic or acute non-optical disease is supervised by the specialist.

● When it is inevitable that serious visual disability exists or will develop early, contact with statutory voluntary agencies catering for handicap is essential.

● There is growing awareness of the need for prophylaxis in ophthalmology. The non-specialist can contribute to better eye health by counselling patients on avoidance of infection and trauma.

21   Ocular therapies

The range of drugs in common use in ophthalmology is not enormous, but it is helpful to consider them separately so that their therapeutic objectives, modes of action and side-effects may be examined.

Some of the ocular side-effects of drugs given for general disease are noted on pages 210–11.

COMMONLY USED EYEDROPS

Most eyedrops fall into a few well-defined groups. The principal categories are:

- Pupil-active drugs
- Anti-inflammatory agents; steroids and others
- Anti-infective agents
- Local anaesthetics
- Placebos.

Administration of eye drops is shown in Figure 21.1.

Pupil-active drugs

These drugs are subdivided into those that enlarge the pupil, mydriatics, and those that constrict the pupil, miotics.

Mydriatics produce their effect by:

- a parasympatholytic reaction, paralysis of the pupil sphincter

- a sympathomimetic action, dilator stimulation.

The best known parasympatholytic drugs are:

Atropine (0.5 or 1 per cent)

Its weaker analogue homatropine (2 per cent)

The shorter-acting synthetic parasympatholytics such as tropicamide (1 per cent) or cyclopentolate (0.5 or 1 per cent).

The effects of atropine act for a long time (often up to a week) after a single instillation; the duration of the action of the other drugs is shorter, perhaps only one or two days.

The short-acting drugs are frequently used for diagnostic dilatation of the pupil. The powerful atropine is reserved for severe cases of corneal inflammation and for iritis where it is important to breakdown adhesions (posterior synechiae) between iris and lens.

An invariable accompaniment of pupil dilatation produced by parasympatholytic drugs is paralysis of accommodation (cycloplegia). It is

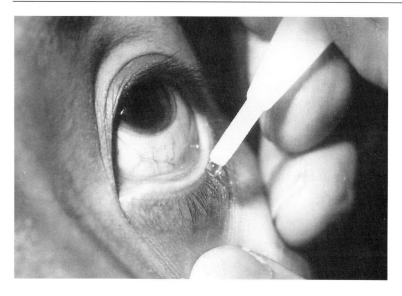

Figure 21.1   Instillation of eyedrops. The lower lid is slid away to make a trough between it and the globe. The eyedrop is applied to the eye from the front while the patient looks upwards. No 'dropping' action is required. It will simply jump in without the dropper end touching the lid.

for this reason that blurred close vision is a frequent complaint of patients who have been given these eyedrops.

The paralysis of accommodation may be intentional when used in refraction (see Chapter 6). Here the pupils are dilated so that the fundi may be inspected, the associated absence of accommodation allowing measurement of an unvarying optical state. In children whose accommodation is very active, it is usual to give atropine drops, or ointment (1 per cent) for a few days (for example, three times a day for three days, or twice a day for a week), before a refraction examination. Over the age of seven years, cyclopentolate or tropicamide will suffice, and can be given at the initial examination, with full effect taking place within the hour.

Another important use of these drugs is in the preoperative and postoperative management of cataract and following glaucoma drainage operations. Before cataract surgery, it is mandatory to produce a widely dilated pupil if extracapsular extraction is planned. A frequently used combination is cyclopentolate (1 per cent) with the sympathomimetic phenylephrine (10 per cent— see below). Cyclopentolate is also extensively used in cataract patients as part of the treatment of postoperative uveitis.

Sympathomimetic pupil dilatation is rarely used on its own, though it is often used in combination with parasympatholytic paralysis. Besides phenylephrine (2.5 or 10 per cent), the two other main drugs considered here are cocaine (2 or 4 per cent), which is of course most

commonly used for its local anaesthetic properties (see page 206), and adrenaline. The latter
is now mainly used in chronic simple glaucoma
(where pupillary dilatation is immaterial) in a 0.5
or 1 per cent strength. Adrenaline in a 0.1 per
cent solution is used to constrict superficial blood
vessels preoperatively. Very weak dilutions are
incorporated in irrigation solutions used in cataract surgery to help keep the pupil dilated.

The vasoconstricting effect of the drugs in this
group is often used in cosmetic 'eye whitening'
preparations. Naphazoline, xylometazoline hydrochloride and phenylephrine are among the
most common found.

Miotics These parasympathomimetic drugs
have already been reviewed in Chapter 13. They
include:

Pilocarpine (0.5 to 4 per cent)
Physostigmine (0.25 to 1 per cent)
Neostigmine methylsulphate (3 per cent)
Carbachol (0.5 per cent)
Phospholine iodide (0.03 to 0.125 per cent).

It was noted that if the patient still has some
accommodative power, this may be disturbed by
a spasm of the ciliary muscle when these drugs
are used.

Therapeutic use of this action is deliberately
sought in accommodative convergent strabismus
in children (see Chapter 19). Here miotics are
used to reduce the child's own need to induce
accommodation, and hence the tendency to
over-converge the eyes.

Glaucoma patients who remain on long-term
miotic therapy may complain of a dimness in
their vision, especially in poorly lit surroundings. This is of course a consequence of the
failure of the pupils to dilate naturally.

Miosis produced by antisympathomimetic
drugs is of no clinical significance.

Other drugs affecting the autonomic nervous
systems are used in the management of chronic
simple glaucoma and are fully discussed in
Chapter 13.

Anti-inflammatory agents

Steroids in common use today are, in order of
increasing effectiveness:

1 Prednisolone drops (0.5 per cent)

2 Fluorometholone drops (0.1 per cent)

3 Betamethasone (0.1 per cent) drops and also
as ointment

4 Clobetasone butyrate drops (0.1 per cent)

5 Dexamethasone drops (0.1 per cent), and
also as ointment.

The principal indications for these anti-
inflammatory drops are:

● Non-infective inflammatory eye disease of
the anterior uvea, including post-operative
uveitis

● Allergic conjunctivitis and blepharitis

● Some forms of keratitis, usually not ulcera-
tive.

Steroid drops should never be given alone for
dendritic ulceration (superficial keratitis caused
by the herpes simplex virus), although combinations of steroids with antiviral agents are
needed for the deep keratitis which occasionally
complicates this. The use of steroids is acceptable
only under the close scrutiny of the ophthalmologist.

All topical steroids may cause the ocular
pressure to rise and the more potent the steroids,
the more this is likely. Newer steroids such as
fluorometholone or clobetasone are said to be
therapeutically potent but less liable to raise eye
pressure. It is also said that prolonged use of
steroids locally may lead to formation of cataract.
This is extremely rare and is far more liable to
occur following systemic steroid therapy over a
long period (see page 89).

The reputation of steroids for spreading infections is probably exaggerated as far as topical use
is concerned; however, the stricture with regard

to herpes simplex remains important (see Chapter 8). This may also apply to chlamydial infections. Here topical steroids, if used at all, should be accompanied by the appropriate anti-infective agent. Combinations of steroids with anti-infective agents, particularly with the antibiotic neomycin, are widespread in other conditions, although the advantage is not clear unless the diagnosis cannot be confirmed.

Non-steroidal anti-inflammatory agents

An important and individual non-steroidal anti-flammatory drug that is of particular value in allergic external eye disease is sodium cromoglycate (2 per cent). Antihistamines typically given with a vasoconstrictor (xylometazoline hydrochloride 0·05 per cent – vasoconstrictor – with antazoline sulphate 0.5 per cent – antihistamine) are also helpful for allergic inflammation.

Anti-infective agents

The commonest type of drops used in chemotherapy are antibiotics: chloramphenicol, neomycin (each 0.5 per cent), and the related soframycin, the tetracyclines and the sulphonamides, particulary sulphacetamide (10 or 30 per cent), as well as antiviral agents.

Acute bacterial infections of the outer eye (conjunctivitis, styes, some types of blepharitis) respond to local antibiotics given frequently (hourly or two hourly).

Chlamydial infection requires a prolonged period of treatment with local sulphonamide drops or tetracycline, as well as systemic oxytetracycline (250 mg four times daily) for three weeks.

Viral infections of the outer eye are often self-limiting and the associated inflammation may be reduced by steroids, provided it is certain that herpes simplex is not responsible (see above).

If herpes simplex is confirmed or suspected to be present, specific antiherpetic agents are now available. These include idoxuridine, cytosine arabinocide, trifluorothymidine and acyclovir. The last of these has the remarkable property of being activated solely in the presence of the herpes virus itself.

In herpes zoster, both antiviral and local steroid therapy will probably be required. Idoxuridine in dimethyl sulphoxide is applied to the skin lesion in the early stages. Acyclovir (locally or systemically) may be helpful but, in any case affecting the globe proper, local steroids are mandatory.

Local anaesthetics

Anaesthetic eyedrops in common use are:

Amethocaine (1 per cent)

Oxybuprocaine (0.4 per cent)

Lignocaine (4 per cent).

These are shorter lasting and less powerful than cocaine, but are sufficient for simple procedures such as removal of corneal foreign bodies or ocular pressure measurement by contact methods. They are also used for operative procedures of a short duration such as glaucoma surgery.

The classical cocaine (1 to 4 per cent strength) is the most powerful, three or four drops at five minute intervals usually being effective in anaesthetizing the outer eye. Cocaine has, however, the possible disadvantages of dilating the pupil and producing a slightly toxic effect, leading to drying of the corneal epithelium.

Cocaine's addictive properties restrict its very wide use, but it remains an important aid to major anterior segment eye surgery carried out under local anaesthesia.

Placebos

Placebo eyedrops have appeared mainly in response to the commonly presenting clinical picture of the general irritation, with or without slight congestion of the outer eye, with no other physical ocular signs present. The whole symptom complex consists of gritty, itchy, hot, dry or wet, painful, red, sore and tender globes combined with a foreign body sensation and a conviction that various previously unnoticed anatomical abnormalities (prominent lacrimal punctum or caruncle, or a slightly prominent lacrimal gland), portend imminent ocular dissolution and blindness. Few if any signs accompany a long and often shifting catalogue of complaints. Sympathetic attempts to explain the true psychosomatic basis of such cases are usually fruitless.

Placebos commonly used are:

Artificial tears, typically hypromellose drops (0.3 per cent), a methylcellulose solution which is also used for genuine cases of reduced lacrimal secretion (see page 142)

Astringents (zinc sulphate)

Vasoconstrictors (see page 135)

Mild chemotherapeutic agents such as propamidine

Antibiotics

Possibly steroids.

The last two cannot be said to be entirely harmless; as noted, the steroid drugs should not be used unsupervised for long periods. The prolonged use of antibiotics is one cause of drop allergy. Combinations of steroids and antibiotics given for no very satisfactory reason are obviously undesirable.

Drop allergy

The common factor in drop allergy is extended exposure to the offending drug. Antibiotics such as chloramphenicol and neomycin are widely prescribed, and repeated exposure may lead to an allergic response. The clinical picture (see Chapter 17) is of an eczematous swelling and inflammation of the eyelids, combined with conjunctival injection.

Some anti-glaucoma preparations, particularly adrenaline and guanethidine, are prone to produce similar reactions; pilocarpine less frequently.

The classical atropine allergy is still occasionally seen, but is now much rarer because diseases such as iritis, which used to be managed by prolonged atropinization, are effectively abbreviated by the use of steroids.

Very occasionally a patient will have an allergic reaction to the preservative in an eyedrop. These are substances in minute concentration intended to keep eyedrops sterile. The whole basis of this branch of therapeutics is somewhat uncertain, and the precise purpose for these chemicals being incorporated is not entirely clear. It seems doubtful that they are 'preserving' anything chemically; and as anti-infective agents not only is their efficacy in question but also the necessity for their inclusion, if the patient concerned is the sole user.

A similarly illogical view seems to have inspired the instruction on drop bottle labels not to use the drops 'X' days after opening. Glaucoma patients in particular often obey this injunction slavishly and go without necessary treatment if a fresh supply of drops is not readily available. The stringencies on use of drops after a precise date are unnecessarily rigid, costly and possibly harmful at times.

LOCAL THERAPY OTHER THAN BY DROPS

This includes:

- Ointments
- Subconjunctival injection
- Retrobulbar injection
- Eyebaths.

Ointments

Ointment may be used as an alternative to drops. Some patients find it easier to use ointments rather than to instil eyedrops. Their therapeutic effect may be more enduring and some agents such as tetracycline, which is not easily water soluble, can be more satisfactorily delivered by this method. Ointments may produce a greasy film over the cornea that may temporarily blur the vision.

Subconjunctival injection

Subconjunctival injections (Figure 21.2) are used to deliver large doses of antibiotics, steroids or other agents in acute situations such as a very severe iritis or keratitis with ulceration, due to a pyogenic infection.

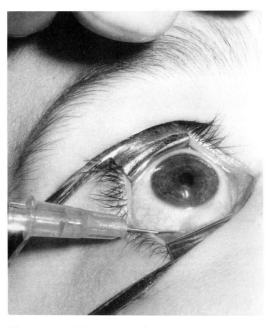

Figure 21.2   Subconjunctival injection.

Subconjunctival injection is also used prophylactically after major ophthalmic surgery, where a common combination might be dexamethasone (4 mg) with soframycin (250 mg). Antibiotics are given by this route for postoperative infections of a dangerous degree.

Subconjunctival injections are given only by an ophthalmologist or trained eye nurse.

Retrobulbar injection

Delivery of a drug into the muscle cone is the classical method of deep local anaesthesia of the eye. All the nerves and the ciliary ganglion are contained within the cone formed by the rectus muscles and the fascia between them, with the globe itself as the 'base' of the cone (see Figure 21.3).

Lignocaine (1 or 2 per cent strengths) is commonly used and 1/200,000 adrenaline may be included.

Although there are also blood vessels within the muscle cone, the procedure of delivering therapeutic agents to the posterior structures of the eye by retrobulbar injection is not well substantiated. However if that is what is required, then systemic therapy should be considered.

Occasionally retobulbar injection causes a haemorrhage with sudden proptosis of the eye. If this occurs preoperatively, the proposed procedure has to be postponed for a few days until the protrusion has subsided.

Eyebaths

Self-medication by eyebaths, though it may be hallowed by the elevated-sounding term inunction, has no serious place in ocular therapeutics.

SYSTEMIC THERAPY

Systemic chemotherapy is required for the following conditions:

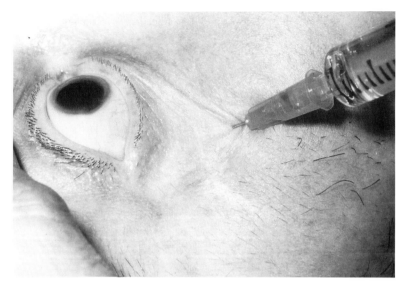

Figure 21.3 Retrobulbar injection.

• Fulminating corneal ulceration by pneumo-coccus or pseudomonas, for example

• Deep ocular infections

• Endophthalmitis resulting from trauma aris-ing postoperatively or from a metastatic source

• Extensive pyogenic infections of the eyelids, lacrimal apparatus or orbit.

The ocular penetration of various antibiotics needs to be considered along with the micro-biological report of the identity and sensitivity of the pathogens. Speed is of the essence, and antibiotics together with steroids (the latter to minimize destructive inflammation) are given immediately, without waiting for laboratory reports. Large oral doses of sodium fusidate (500 mg three times daily) are said to be valuable in this situation. The penicillins, tetracyclines, erythromycin and even chloramphenicol are considered.

In suspected bacterial endophthalmitis, it is usual to combine local chemotherapy and ster-oids with systemic medication. In addition to eyedrops, frequent (even daily) subconjunctival injections are given which contain, typically, an aminoglycoside, a penicillin derivative and dexamethasone. Treatment becomes even more complex if external cultures of the eye, or of aspirated vitreous specimens, show the presence of fungi (as is not uncommon).

Systemic steroid therapy is sometimes employed in cases where the response to local steroids is inadequate. For example, a very severe anterior uveitis, spontaneous or postoperative, may require this type of therapy. If steroid therapy is necessary for posterior uveitis, it can be effective only if it is given systemically. The combined use of systemic chemotherapy and steroids is helpful in specific infections such as toxoplasmosis affecting the posterior segment of the eye.

Typically, prednisolone in an enteric-coated form is given in doses of up to 40 mg a day. Larger doses are sometimes indicated as primary therapy for cranial arteritis, or in dysthyroid eye disease.

Other important ocular therapies delivered systemically include acetazolamide in glaucoma and pyrimethamine for toxoplasmosis.

Ocular toxicology

An enormous number of systemically administered drugs may affect the eye, and a full catalogue of them would be out of place here. However, some do require special mention and are discussed below.

Functional effects

Drugs with an activity which either principally or secondarily affect the autonomic nervous system, particularly with parasympatholytic activity, may interfere with accommodation and cause blurring of near vision. Many drugs in this group may cause slight pupillary dilatation and are therefore to be avoided in cases of closed angle glaucoma.

Some antihypertensive agents can cause blurring of the vision. This may be due to their autonomic effect or possibly to temporary retinal ischaemia during general vascular readjustment.

The opposite condition of spasm of accommodation is rare, but this can lead to temporary short-sightedness; sulphonamides and acetazolamide have been noted as causing this.

Structural effects

Corneal changes occur in patients on prolonged treatment with anti-malarials; the use of chloroquine in rheumatoid arthritis falls into this category. Wispy, sheaf-like infiltrates occur in the cornea, giving rise in some patients to the appearance of haloes around lights.

It is uncommon for there to be corneal involvement of any significant consequence and, even when the signs are visible by slit-lamp examination, there may be no symptoms at all. The retinal toxicity of chloroquine is quite another matter and the drug should be withdrawn immediately on detection of the condition.

Amiodarone used in cardiac arrhythmias produces an identical corneal infiltration but not, it is believed, any retinal damage.

Toxic cataract is a possible complication in patients taking systemic steroids over a prolonged period (Figure 21.14). It is not otherwise

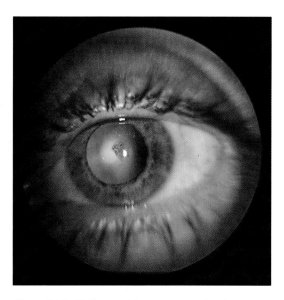

Figure 21.4   Early steroid cataract seen by the ophthalmoscope.

commonly seen in modern therapeutics. In many patients there is no possibility of withdrawal of steroids, as they are life-preserving, and if the lens opacity becomes sufficiently disabling, cataract surgery is undertaken. Usually the risks of surgery are related only to the patient's general condition and age.

The possible side-effects of steroids locally administered have been mentioned elsewhere— rise in intraocular pressure, aggravation and even recrudescence of herpes simplex keratitis.

Retinal damage may occur from many systemic sources. The anti-malarials (particularly chloro-quine) have unpredictably serious effects in some patients when given over prolonged periods for rheumatoid arthritis.

Typically, a macular pigmentary change occurs in a bull's-eye target arrangement, thus interfering with central vision. Eventually the rest of the retina becomes affected and a picture not unlike retinitis pigmentosa develops, with severe loss of field of vision. The condition, if advanced, is irreversible.

Its early diagnosis is facilitated by regular check-ups of vision, colour vision and visual fields. It may also be helped by electrophysi-ological tests, in particular there may be a reduction in the electro-oculogram (EOG), which is believed to be an indication of retinal pigment epithelial function. This is somewhat different from the electroretinogram (ERG) and is a potential of about 6 mV, the cornea being electroposi-tive relative to the retina. The eye is therefore something of a dipole and potential changes can be recorded by electrodes being placed at the sides.

The classical anti-malarial quinine, if taken in excess, may produce sudden blindness with a picture, often bilateral, rather like central retinal artery occlusion.

Psychotropic drugs may also lead to macular pigmentation and loss of vision, but only after prolonged, very high dosage.

Ethambutol, an important anti-tuberculous drug, may be a cause of visual loss presumed to be at least partially retinotoxic in nature. Loss of acuity, disturbed colour vision and the development of field defects are typical features. Fortunately, if discovered early, withdrawal of the drug will lead to a complete recovery.

Toxic neuropathy of the optic nerve is uncommon. The classical affection resulting from the smoking of pipe shag tobacco (tobacco/alcohol amblyopia) leads to a loss of vision with characteristic paracentral scotomata (blind spots), particularly to red objects. It is believed to result from the inadequate detoxication of cyanide in the blood stream, a function in which vitamin B_{12} plays a significant role. Treatment is by hydroxo-cobalamin injections.

Optic atrophy   A much more severe and irreversible optic atrophy may result from methyl-alcohol ingestion. Subconjunctival and retinal haemorrhages may occur in patients on anti-coagulant therapy.

The management of iatrogenic toxicity

This should of course be prophylactic. Patients on those therapies that have known ocular side-effects should be monitored closely. This particularly applies to the drugs mentioned above.

There appear to be no conclusive pointers as to which patients taking these drugs will suffer side-effects. Nevertheless, early detection may prompt withdrawal of the offending drug, perhaps leading to recovery. Failing this, there is at least a chance of averting the full progression of the toxic effect.

PRACTICAL POINTS

● Among the most common ophthalmic drugs are the pupil-active mydriatics and miotics. Mydriatics are used in diagnosis, in refraction, in corneal disease, in uveitis and postoperatively in many conditions.

● Miotics are principally used in glaucoma. They are also used in accommodative convergent strabismus in children.

● The topical steroids are used in non-infective disorders of the outer eye. They may produce raised intra-orbital pressure. Although their propensity to spread infection is probably exaggerated, they must be avoided in herpes simplex infection.

● Infections of the outer eye are normally treated with topical antibiotics.

● Placebo eyedrops may be of value to patients with longstanding psychosomatic problems.

● Subconjunctival and retrobulbar injections are used where very intensive local administration of drugs is indicated.

● Systemic chemotherapy is used in fulminating corneal ulceration, deep ocular infections and postoperative or traumatic endophthalmitis as well as in severe infections of the neighbouring structures.

● Drugs used in other conditions may affect vision; antihypertensive agents can cause blurring and antirheumatic drugs may produce corneal and retinal changes. Toxic cataract can occur from the prolonged use of systemic steroids.

Cardiovascular disease and diabetes

The ophthalmology dealt with in Part 2 had little direct connection with the human body as a whole. Those terms such as cataract, glaucoma and detachment belong to the subject of ophthalmology as a 'closed' specialty. In the remainder of Part 3 we examine the relationship between ophthalmology and other branches of medicine.

It is a prevailing view that there is an ophthalmic complication or sign for almost every general medical disease, and that all eye conditions are associated in some way with general health. This is not the case, however. The bulk of the eye specialist's work is concerned with conditions that have little discernible relationship with general medical disease.

Nevertheless, the eye specialist, preoccupied as he or she is with such disorders, will be particularly on the alert for the minority of clinical conditions in which there is just such a relationship. It is with those relatively few general diseases that have major ophthalmic implications that this and the succeeding chapters are concerned.

Retinal vascular disease

Retinal vascular disease is a major association of certain life-threatening conditions. We therefore examine this first, under the following headings:

- Obstruction of major retinal vessels

- Vascular retinopathies: arteriosclerotic, hypertensive and diabetic.

Pathology of the retinal blood vessels is important from two standpoints:

1 It may produce disturbance of vision or of the visual fields

2 It may give evidence, even without symptoms, of vascular diseases of a more widespread nature.

If acute symptoms are present, they often point to a **retinal vascular accident** of some type or other. If there are no symptoms, or there is a slowly developing history, the ophthalmic picture is referred to as a **vascular retinopathy**. Any retinopathy may of course have a vascular accident imposed upon it or may be complicated by other acute episodes such as a vitreous haemorrhage.

Consequently, for every physician concerned with arteriosclerotic disease, vascular hypertension or diabetes mellitus, an inspection of the retina is an essential part of the general clinical examination. It goes without saying that whoever inspects the fundus, for whatever reason (even during a sight test for spectacles, for example), vascular changes that may have implications for the patient's general health must be sought.

Retinal vascular accidents

The arrangements of the retinal vessels is important in understanding their pathology. The arterial supply (the central artery) is a branch of the ophthalmic artery, itself a branch of the internal carotid. It enters the optic nerve a short distance behind the eyeball to emerge into the eye on the optic disc and immediately divides into upper and lower main branches. Each of these then splits into nasal and temporal subdivisions which spread out, with further branching on the inner retinal surface, to extend out to the periphery (Figure 22.1).

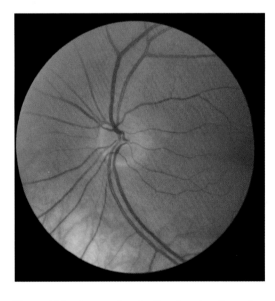

Figure 22.1 A normal optic disc showing the pattern of emerging vessels. There is a physiological cup present as well as a small temporal crescent.

There are no significant anastomoses between the central retinal circulation and any other vessels; the artery is therefore effectively an end artery. The capillaries of this circulation supply only the inner layers of the retina; the outer retina, including the pigment epithelium and the rods and cones, is nourished from the capillary bed of the choroid circulation just outside it. The main superior temporal and inferior temporal branches of the central artery above and below the macula send arterioles towards, but not actually reaching, the macula itself.

The veins in this system collect as tributaries parallel to the arterial circulation, eventually forming the central retinal vein. This leaves the eye near to the central artery but has an uncertain and variable termination in relation to the orbital veins which are themselves of no predictable pattern, sometimes ending in the pterygoid plexus via the inferior orbital vein.

The self-contained nature of the retinal vasculature is an important factor to consider when studying the effects of an obstruction. The way the vessels subdivide is also relevant as such an obstruction may affect a central vessel or one or more of its branches or tributaries.

Obstruction of major retinal vessels is discussed under the following categories:

- Central retinal artery occlusion
- Branch arterial occlusion
- Intermittent arterial occlusion
- Central retinal vein occlusion
- Tributary occlusion of the retinal veins.

Central retinal artery occlusion is an uncommon but important clinical event which presents as a sudden, painless loss of vision; almost invariably in one eye only. The blindness is usually virtually complete, with light perception lost due to all the inner retinal layers being functionless. The pupil fails to react directly to light, although its consensual reaction is normal. The fundus is easily seen and shows threadlike or invisible arterioles and a static and broken up venous

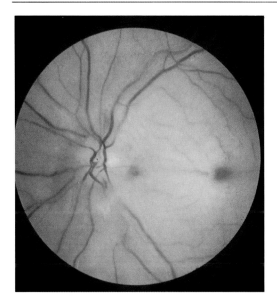

Figure 22.2 Classical central retinal artery occlusion with cherry red spot.

column, in which the small segments of the blood shift back and forth, an appearance known as 'cattle trucking'. There is a whitening of the retina around the macula with, in classical cases, a cherry red spot appearing at the macula itself (Figure 22.2). The red spot may simply be the choroidal red reflex seen through the thinned and therefore less whitened retina at the macula.

Causes

The three causes of central retinal artery occlusion are spasm, thrombosis and embolus. Spasm alone cannot easily be distinguished from the effects of thrombosis. Embolism may be indicated by the presence of a glistening cholesterol plaque on the disc in the central retinal artery.

Treatment

The condition must be treated as an emergency, dictated by the fact that retinal ischaemia lasting for more than a few hours is followed by irrecoverable loss of vision. The following points are of particular importance:

1 Any patient with a sudden loss of vision will need immediate specialist clinical advice. In such cases the measures taken to restore the circulation aim to dilate the retinal blood vessels both directly and, by softening the eyes, indirectly. A simple first-aid way of achieving the latter is to rub the eye for ten seconds, stop for ten seconds, and repeat four or five times. This can be done initially by the patient. Pressing on the eye expels aqueous humour and reduces pressure, leaving a softened eye.

2 The ophthalmologist gives a retrobulbar injection of a vasodilator drug such as acetylcholine, tolazoline or praxilene, and an intravenous injection of acetazolamide. Paracentesis of the anterior chamber is usually performed to expel aqueous humour. This last manoeuvre produces a sudden drop in eye pressure and can cause the retinal vasculature to expand and break down a possible spasm, which in any case complicates both thrombosis and embolism.

3 An erythrocyte sedimentation rate (ESR) should be performed on the grounds that arteritis may be present, and steroids and anticoagulants are sometimes administered; steroids are advisable if the ESR is very high.

Unfortunately, treatment is often unsuccessful either because of the basic irreversibility of the pathology (thrombosis, for example) or because of death of retinal cells. Although the retinal circulation may be restored, vision is often only partially restored in some field, the central vision being lost. Occasionally an embolus is swept into the periphery of the arterial circulation, and there is a reasonable return of central vision.

Consultation with a general physician on the systemic vascular state or possible embolic

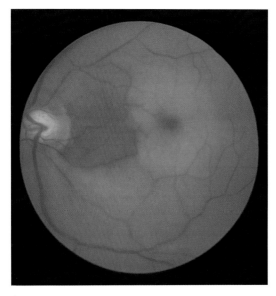

a

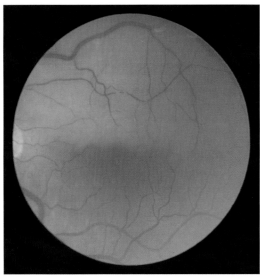

b

Figure 22.3 Partial occlusions of the retinal arterial circulation: (*a*) shows a central artery occlusion with sparing of the papillo-macular area because of a patent cilioretinal artery. (*b*) shows the effect of occlusion of the upper main branch of the central artery. Oedema of the macula is present, which is sharply divided by a horizontal line from the normal retina below.

sources, such as the heart or the carotids, is essential.

Branch arterial occlusion has several effects. Even when the central retinal artery is involved, the central vision may be unaffected owing to an independent unobstructed macular arterial supply, a ·cilioretinal artery (Figure 22.3a). Sometimes this vessel alone is obstructed, affecting only the central vision and leaving the remainder of the retina normally vascularized.

Sometimes only one of the four main branches of the artery is affected (Figure 22.3b). If the temporal branch of the upper or lower main division is affected, the macula may suffer and a corresponding field loss results, the central vision being split, and the dividing line often astonishingly sharp between the seeing and non-seeing area. Such sharp half-divisions are reminiscent of the hemianopia of neurology; although these are usually vertical, whereas the retinal vascular pattern dictates that partial field loss caused by retinal ischaemia is always horizontal.

The causes and treatment of these branch occlusions are the same as for central artery occlusion.

Intermittent arterial occlusion This is the ocular effect of the general medical condition of transient ischaemic attacks (TIAs). The effect of emboli on the general retinal arterial circulation sometimes spontaneously resolves because the embolus moves into a more peripheral part of the retinal vascular tree, and then fragments (Figure 22.4). In so doing, it may cause an intermittent blindness, producing a pattern of field loss dictated by the subdivision of the retinal vessels. Thus, a patient may complain of the lower field being lost, followed by the upper field, with resultant complete blindness for a short period; recovery eventually begins in the upper field.

Similar TIAs are thought to arise even in the absence of emboli if an already diseased retinal circulation is further embarrassed by a temporary drop of systemic blood pressure.

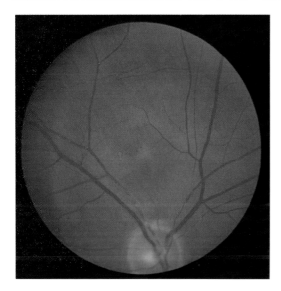

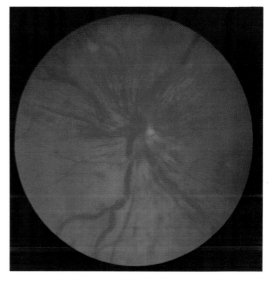

Figure 22.4   Multiple emboli in the retinal arteries.

Figure 22.5   Central retinal vein thrombosis.

In all cases, particular attention should be paid to any history of temporary neurological episodes on the opposite side of the body, as well as to the state of the carotids. The management of carotid occlusion is beyond the scope of this book, but it is common in milder cases for aspirin to be given by mouth over long periods.

Central retinal vein occlusion   This is almost always thrombotic and slower to develop than the conditions discussed above. The loss of vision is profound, although not quite as complete as in arterial occlusion. The retinal picture is of plum-coloured, dilated and tortuous veins emerging from a swollen optic disc. Numerous haemorrhages lie alongside these veins, from the optic disc to far out into the periphery (Figure 22.5).

The cause is sometimes unidentifiable, there being no history of general vascular disease. However, associated diabetes or hypertension are quite commonly found.

Prognosis

There is no effective treatment for an established occlusion of the central vein or of its tributaries. Occasionally, some months after a central vein occlusion, glaucoma will develop in the already near-blind eye. This presents acutely with redness and pain, the cause being the development of a vascular membrane on the front of the iris, 'rubeosis', and over the angle of the anterior chamber. Laser treatment of the retina may prevent or abort this development. However, once it has occurred, complex surgery may be indicated to reduce the pressure. The success of such a procedure, as well as of medical treatment, is questionable. Although many such blind and painful eyes can be made comfortable by the retrobulbar injection of alcohol, others require surgical removal.

Tributary occlusion of the retinal veins   This may be symptomless and noted only at a routine fundus examination; when, for example, superior temporal tributary occlusion affecting the macula may be found. However, the associated haemorrhages and retinal oedema mask the sensory elements to some extent so that the patient notices the central vision is affected (Figure 22.6). If the haemorrhages clear away

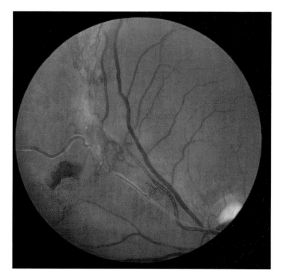

Figure 22.7   The late effects of a vascular occlusion. Vessel sheathing and neovascular formations are visible.

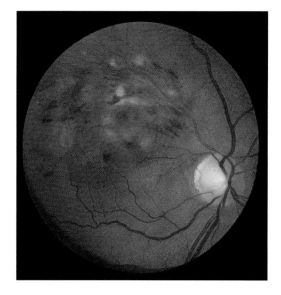

Figure 22.6   A superior temporal venous tributary occlusion.

and the ischaemic damage to the central retina is not severe, some improvement in vision will occur.

After a time, all signs of the venous occlusion, whether central or tributary, may disappear from the retina, possibly as a result of recanalization. The vein may appear sheathed and knots of new vessels or collaterals may develop (Figure 22.7). The former may bleed and, to prevent this, laser coagulation may be indicated. The disc may become pale once the oedema has subsided.

Some but not all of these vascular accidents, either venous or arterial, are related to pre-existing retinal vascular pathologies that may be symptomless. We now turn to these vascular retinopathies.

Vascular retinopathies

Three clinical pictures are common: arteriosclerosis, hypertension and diabetes. Arteriosclerosis, as an aging phenomenon, may occur together with either of the other two conditions.

As noted, all retinopathies may be symptomless unless there is a direct involvement of the macula or some vascular accident occurs.

Arteriosclerosis

A very marked arteriosclerosis may occur in the retinal vessels and be discovered during a routine eye inspection. Its presence may confirm a widespread involvement of the blood vessels, already the cause of a systemic disorder such as a stroke.

The retinal arteries show a combination of narrowing irregularity and tortuosity, with altered reflexes from their walls which are variously described as 'silver wiring' or 'copper wiring' (Figure 22.8). The reflex is due to increased visibility of the vessel wall, which is normally transparent. Lengths of the vessels may occasionally appear like threads of cotton, while other segments may show sheathing along the walls. The veins may be little altered, but show changes at the arteriovenous crossing (nipping). In simple arteriosclerotic changes, haemorrhages or exudates are insignificant features of the clinical picture.

If parts of the retina are ischaemic, field constriction corresponding to the affected areas will be found. If extensive retinal ischaemia is present, the central vision may fail and the optic disc become pale.

Arteriosclerotic disease of the choroid is discussed more fully in Chapter 12 and is responsible for one particular form of senile macular degeneration, the variety known as choroidal sclerosis.

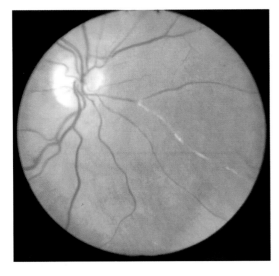

Figure 22.8 Sheathing and silver wiring of the retinal arteriole.

Hypertensive retinopathy

The presentation of this condition varies according to the speed of development and severity of the hypertension, its cause and the presence or absence of any pre-existing retinal arterial disease.

In benign essential hypertension, there are, according to convention, four progressive stages of involvement of the retina and its vessels:

- **Stages One and Two** are the narrowing of the arterial calibre and arteriovenous crossing changes. Diagnosis at these stages is complicated since appearances may be incidental aging phenomena, while in younger subjects the narrowing may be due to spasm rather than structural shrinkage of arterial size. Arteriovenous nipping, perhaps with obstruction of the vein behind the crossing and with banking is a frequent association of hypertension, although it can occur without it (Figure 22.9). These stages are usually symptomless.

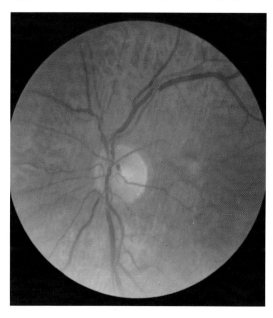

Figure 22.9 Nipping of the retinal veins. The veins are constricted at the first arteriovenous crossings of both the upper and lower temporal arterioles.

● **Stages Three and Four** are the presence of haemorrhages and exudates and finally oedema of the disc, sometimes associated with oedema of the macula.

Haemorrhages and exudates are usually symptomless unless a vitreous haemorrhage occurs or the deposits involve the macula. Even the final stage may occur in patients free of any ocular complaint.

However, if the condition has arisen quickly (accelerated or malignant hypertension) or the condition is longstanding, visual symptoms do quite frequently occur. Occasionally flashes of light are experienced, or an intermittent loss of vision is experienced, which is due to spasm of the arterioles.

With significant macular oedema there is sustained depression of vision. It should be remembered that visual symptoms may also arise from cortical involvement in hypertensive encephalopathy.

In a florid hypertensive retinopathy, there may be macular oedema, scattered, numerous haemorrhages (many flame-shaped as they lie in the nerve fibre of the retina) and soft and hard exudates, the last of these often radiating from the macula, a star figure (Figures 22.10 and 22.11).

The presence of soft exudates (cotton wool spots) in particular are evidence of the severity of the condition, as they represent focal ischaemic change due to localized closure of retinal capillaries.

The finding of such a retinal picture, even without, but especially with, visual deterioration, is a strong indication to reduce the blood pressure with the appropriate regimen. The whole retinal appearance may resolve in a few weeks and vision will return to normal unless, as occasionally happens, the spasm or other obstruction of the circulation in the central retina has led to permanent ischaemic damage.

There is a belief that a true renal retinopathy exists in patients with hypertension associated with end-stage renal failure. The fundus picture is held to be more than that produced by hypertension alone. Others argue that the complex mixture of acute and chronic hypertensive signs can be explained by the clinical variation of the blood pressure and that the severe deterioration of the final picture corresponds to accelerated and severe rises. Nevertheless it is known that renal dialysis, which has saved the lives of so many renal patients, often leads to the lowering of the blood pressure without antihypertensive treatment and, at the same time, to a complete return to normal of the fundus appearance.

It should not be assumed that the retinal changes of hypertension invariably proceed through the four stages outlined above. Occasionally papilloedema may be the only retinal sign. In some cases of severe hypertension there are negligible retinal changes. At any stage a retinal vessel occlusion, especially venous, may supervene; some believe that the

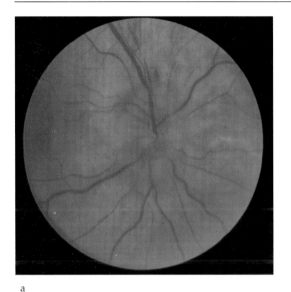

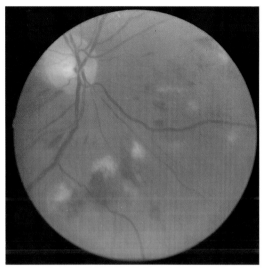

a   b

Figure 22.10   (*a*) Papilloedema and (*b*) retinal
haemorrhage in cases of severe hypertension.

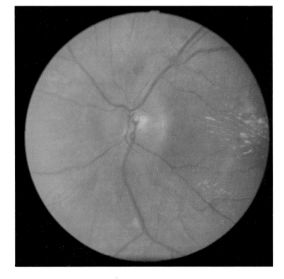

Figure 22.11   A macular fan of exudate in severe
hypertension.

nipping seen ophthalmologically represents a
true venous obstruction predisposing to thrombosis.

The treatment of hypertensive retinopathy
(whether affecting vision or not) is to reduce the
blood pressure to as near normal as possible.
Rapid reduction, although said by some to be
inadvisable on the grounds that a venous thrombosis may be encouraged, is indicated if there is
severe ischaemic macular oedema. Treatment is
in any case the sphere of the cardiovascular
specialist.

Diabetic retinopathy

This is the most important ocular complication of
diabetes and the commonest cause of blindness
in the middle years of life. Its presence may be
discovered sooner in maturity-onset diabetes,
than in younger patients. Clinical symptoms of

the retinopathy are, however, often delayed by up to ten years even in the former group.

The symptoms are either progressive failure of vision owing to a steadily advancing retinopathy involving the macula, or sudden visual loss owing to vitreous haemorrhage, which may or may not clear quickly. Following repeated vitreous haemorrhages, severe loss of sight and blindness may result from detachment of the retina.

The appearances of the retinopathy in diabetes are bewilderingly varied. The following signs may be found:

1 Microaneurysms

2 Haemorrhages in or on the retina, or into the vitreous

3 Hard exudates

4 Macular oedema

5 Cotton wool spots (soft exudates)

6 Neovascularization; new vessel formation on the retina or optic disc

7 Fibro-glial proliferation into the vitreous, retinitis proliferans.

All these changes can be related to abnormalities of the retinal capillaries.

Fluorescein angiography (see page 98) has shown that in many cases there are extensive areas where the capillary bed is closed, leading to retinal anoxia or hypoxia.

Clinical types of diabetic affection of the retina are subdivided into non-proliferative or proliferative, according to the absence or presence of new vessels:

● **Non-proliferative retinopathy** is characterized by microaneurysms, blot haemorrhages and hard exudates and if the macula is not affected, may have little effect on the vision (Figures 22.12 and 22.13). The condition is also known as background retinopathy. If macular

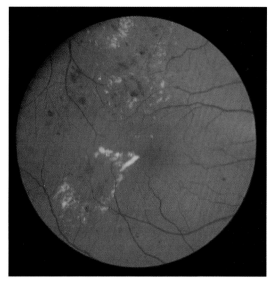

Figure 22.12 Background diabetic retinopathy with a predominance of exudates.

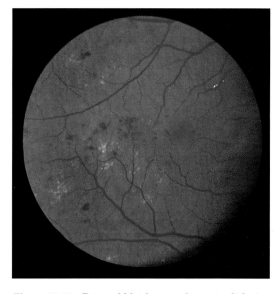

Figure 22.13 Dot and blot haemorrhages in diabetic retinopathy.

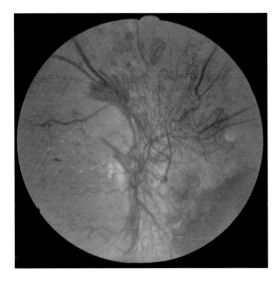

Figure 22.14 An extreme example of new vessel formation affecting both the optic disc and the retina in proliferative diabetic retinopathy.

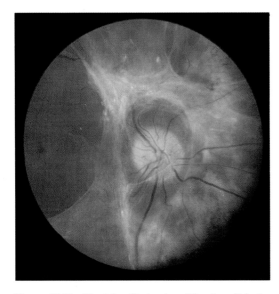

Figure 22.15 The late effects of proliferative diabetic retinopathy.

oedema is present, however, background retinopathy can seriously impair vision.

● **Proliferative retinopathy** is a far more serious condition than that above. New vessels are particularly prone to leakage and this may occur from any, whether intraretinal, epi-retinal or preretinal (Figures 22.14 and 22.15). Extensive bleeding from a preretinal vessel produces preretinal and vitreous haemor-rhages. Eventually the new vessels, which bleed repeatedly into the vitreous, become associated with fibro-glial proliferation, which infiltrates the vitreous structure. Finally, the irregular shrinkage of these glial outgrowths pulls away the retina, the so-called traction retinal detachment. Once this is fairly wide-spread, blindness is almost inevitable.

Treatment of diabetic retinopathy   Control of the diabetes may play a significant part in preventing or delaying the onset of the con-dition. However, once it is established, even excellent control will often not prevent pro-gression, although the rate may be reduced.

The only effective ways of arresting certain types of retinopathy is by photocoagulation, either by xenon arc or by argon laser. The laser is directed at the hypoxic areas of the retina so as to destroy them completely (Figure 22.16). The diseased capillary bed, so treated, becomes anoxic and no longer leaks. The associated microaneurysms are also destroyed and cannot therefore bleed.

In treating background retinopathy affecting the macula, photocoagulation of the affected areas may be necessary very close to the fovea. While treatment is less difficult with the argon laser than with the xenon arc, this type of treatment may be dangerous and great care is essential if the fovea is to be avoided. In any event, the visual improvement, if any, is often unspectacular. If the treated areas are distant from the fovea, however, significant benefit (if only in preventing progression) may result. Non-specific photocoagulation performed in a grid pattern close to the macula, or in a horse-shoe

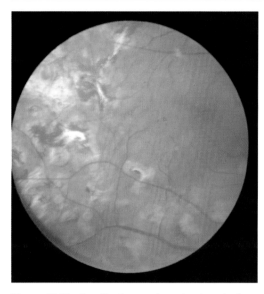

Figure 22.16 Localized argon laser treatment of diabetic maculopathy.

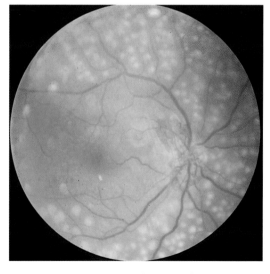

Figure 22.17 The picture of panretinal photocoagulation carried out with the argon laser; multiple white areas of retinal oedema are present. Later these areas are simply replaced by atrophic white scars with pigmentation.

pattern temporal to it, is sometimes helpful in cases of diabetic maculopathy.

The principle of converting hypoxic areas of capillary closure to anoxic scars by photocoagulation is widely applied in proliferative retinopathy, particularly when neovascularization of the optic disc is well developed (Figure 22.17). Here panretinal photocoagulation is carried out, with numerous (up to 3000) small laser burns being made in the periphery of the retina and extending towards, but keeping a suitable distance from, the macula and the optic disc areas.

The technique may also be applied to preventing neovascularization. Fluorescein angiography may indicate many ischaemic areas of capillary closure as possible sites of future new vessel formation. Panretinal photocoagulation to destroy these is therefore indicated.

Finally, photocoagulation is often used to coagulate new vessels that have bled or are likely to bleed into the vitreous.

As noted, the operation of vitrectomy (see page 94) in the treatment of vitreous haemorrhage has a part to play in very advanced proliferative retinopathy.

Other diabetic eye disorders   The sight may be disturbed in diabetes by cataract or by alterations in refraction.

Cataract   Two forms of cataract occur in diabetics, one presenting in the young, unstable diabetic (often with rapid opacification of both lenses) and the other in older patients with a very similar appearance to senile cataract. It may, however, simply be that the aging diabetic is more susceptible to senile cataract.

Myopia   The optical changes that occur in diabetes are particularly important in that the myopia that develops in an untreated and as yet undiagnosed diabetic may be the presenting feature of the whole disease. An eye specialist who encounters myopia that has developed after the age of twenty years would suspect either the onset of diabetes or of a precataractous change in the lens of the eye.

Treatment of the diabetes reverses the myopic tendency; the refractive change is believed to be due to an osmotically determined alteration in hydration rather than opacification of the lens.

Iris neovascularization   Advanced diabetic eye disease may include neovascularization of the front of the iris, and this can lead to an obstruction of the angle of the anterior chamber. The neovascular glaucoma which develops is difficult to treat and is just like thrombotic glaucoma which follows a central retinal vein occlusion (see page 217). Some reduction in iris neovascularization is believed to be produced by panretinal photocoagulation, the treatment for one form of retinopathy (see page 224).

Diabetic patients are also said to be more prone to both iritis and episcleritis (see pages 16–18). Neuropathic complications of diabetes can occasionally present to the ophthalmologist as extrinsic ocular muscle palsies and it is believed that a particular diabetic form of optic neuritis occurs (see Chapter 23).

PRACTICAL POINTS

● Vascular conditions such as arteriosclerotic disease, vascular hypertension and diabetes produce significant ocular changes. Where these conditions are known or suspected, an examination of the retina is essential. The discovery of the characteristic retinopathy associated with these conditions is of great importance in the diagnosis and general management of the patient.

● Central retinal artery occlusion may be due to spasm, thrombosis or embolus. The condition must be treated as an emergency. An immediate first-aid method to restore circulation is to rub the eye for ten-second intervals.

● Branch arterial occlusion can produce sharply demarcated loss of field.

● Intermittent arterial occlusion, transient ischaemic attacks, cause temporary loss of vision and particular attention should be paid to a history of other temporary neurological episodes.

● Central retinal vein occlusion produces a characteristic swollen optic disc with tortuous, plum-coloured veins. There is no effective treatment, and some months after onset glaucoma may also develop.

● It is thought by some that an acute form of retinopathy in hypertensive patients is associated with end-stage renal failure, and this can be reversed by renal dialysis. The blood pressure is lowered and the normal appearance of the fundus is restored.

● Diabetic retinopathy is the commonest cause of blindness in middle life. There is a confusing number of signs. Once diagnosis is confirmed, the condition may possibly be arrested by strict diabetic control and photocoagulation.

23   Neurology and ophthalmology

To appreciate the extent of the inter-relationship between neurology and ophthalmology, we need only remind ourselves of the visual pathway, the oculomotor nerves and the pupil reflexes. The important signs and symptoms of neuro-ophthalmic disease are considered here. The most widely occurring clinical conditions are discussed in Chapter 24.

Presentation and association of neuro-ophthalmic diseases

Two important aspects need to be considered:

1 Neurological disease will occasionally present as an eye problem

2 Associated ophthalmic signs are commonly discovered or looked for during investigation of disorders affecting other parts of the nervous system.

Presenting neuro-ophthalmic symptoms

The presenting symptoms are:

- Loss of vision
- Transient visual disorder
- Field defects
- Diplopia
- Headache
- Flashes of light
- Visual hallucinations.

Loss of vision   A sudden disturbance or loss of vision may occur in acute optic neuritis, ischaemic papillopathy, in sudden compression of the lower visual pathway and in stroke. Slow progressive loss of vision may occur in chronic compression of the lower visual pathway and in longstanding papilloedema resulting from a raised intracranial pressure. It may also occur in certain toxic or infective conditions of the optic nerve (tobacco amblyopia and syphilis). The optic nerve may also suffer in multiple sclerosis.

Transient visual disorder   Recurrent transient loss of vision can be an important presentation of embolic cerebral vascular disease in the form of transient ischaemic attacks (TIAs).

Field defects   Subjectively noticed field defects may occasionally present as a principal complaint. For example, the patient may bump into things or complain that he cannot see objects to the side of his vision.

Diplopia may be a presenting symptom of an affection of any of the nerves or muscles responsible for eye movements. Its differential diagnosis may be difficult, especially in cases where it is intermittent and where pre-existing ocular muscle imbalances are part of the clinical picture.

Headache may present as an eye problem with a query as to its ocular origin. This in turn can lead to the discovery of papilloedema caused by raised intracranial pressure. Pain in the brow or eye itself may be classified as ophthalmic migraine if associated with disturbed muscle balance. The pain of migrainous neuralgia ('cluster headache') is sometimes described as being in the eye.

Flashes of light occasionally occur as a result of cerebral cortical disease, either vascular or neoplastic, and are of course an important feature of migraine. Apart from migraine, however, the causes of flashes of light are much more likely to be ocular.

Hallucinations Formed hallucinatory figures are never ocular in origin. They may signify cortical arterio-sclerotic changes but can be toxic in origin (alcohol, DOPA, for example), or associated with psychiatric disturbances.

Ophthalmic signs associated with neurological disease

The particular features to be considered in a routine neuro-ophthalmological examination are:

- Central vision and the field of vision
- Fundus appearances — the optic discs
- Ocular movements

- Gaze palsies
- Nystagmus
- The pupil
- Proptosis and enophthalmos
- The position and function of the eyelids
- The corneal sensitivity.

The cranial nerves II–VIII and the autonomic system are therefore all relevant.

Central vision and the field of vision   Although a patient with a central visual defect may complain of blurred sight, often a peripheral visual field defect may go unnoticed. Indeed both central visual loss and field defects are important signs of neurological disease, even when there are no other obvious symptoms. These two signs are obviously related. The central vision is affected when there is a defect in the part of the visual field that is subserved by the papillomacular (disc to macula) nerve fibres. These are the axons of the ganglion cells of the macula and they pass to the optic disc to form an important part of the optic nerve. Any severe affection of this 'bundle' leads to a marked loss of central vision with a blind spot or blank patch, known more accurately as a central scotoma.

A scotoma is an isolated, non-seeing island which may occur anywhere in the visual field. It may be undetected, having no effect on the central vision if it is peripheral. A scotoma is of course not necessarily neurologically caused; for instance, a patch of old choroidoretinitis may produce a scotoma in the field of vision.

Neurological causes of field defects, either of the scotomatous type or in the form of contraction of the peripheral field of vision, are legion.

The methods of recording the visual field are outlined in Chapter 13, but it is important to emphasize that a 'neurological' field loss can often be detected by the use of coloured test objects, especially earlier, rather than the standard white ones.

Localization of the pathology in the visual pathway causing the defect is simple and is

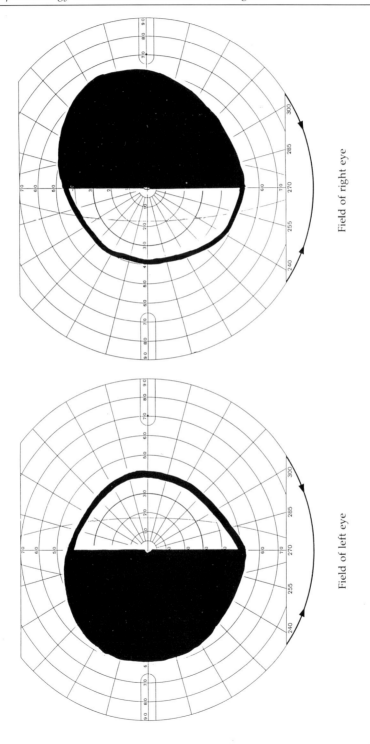

Field of left eye   Field of right eye

Figure 23.1   The fields in a case of bitemporal hemianopia.

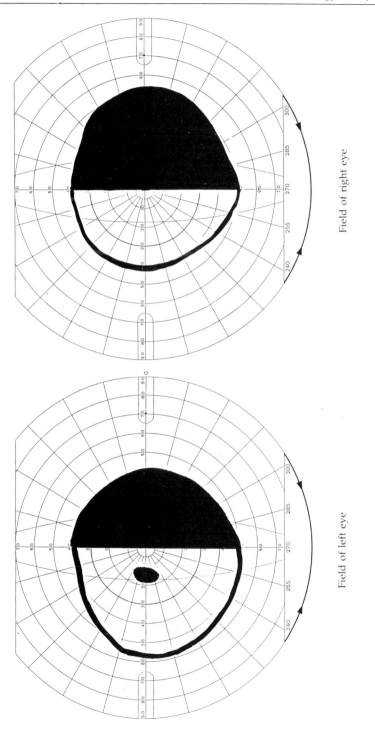

Field of right eye

Field of left eye

Figure 23.2   The fields in a case of right homonymous hemianopia.

based on the anatomy. The key feature is that the fibres of the optic nerve from the basal halves of both retinae, subserving the temporal fields, cross in the chiasma to form part of the optic tract of the opposite side (see Figure 1.4). Orbital lesions affect only one optic nerve and therefore the field of vision of that eye. Intracranial lesions anterior to the chiasma may do likewise, but a space-occupying lesion may also affect the other optic nerve. In such cases, extensive but predominantly temporal field loss of one eye and early temporal loss in the fellow eye are often present. Finally, symmetrical chiasmal compression can produce a complete bitemporal hemianopia (half-vision) (Figure 23.1) or quadrantropia if the pressure is mainly from above or below.

Central to the chiasma, pregeniculate or postgeniculate lesions involve fibres from both eyes and the field defects (scotomatous or larger) are homonymous; that is to say, they involve the same part of the visual field of both eyes. The defects are therefore both in the right or both in the left halves of the fields of vision. Peripheral to the lateral geniculate lesions in the optic tracts tend to produce incongruous homonymous scotomata, the defects in the two fields being unequal in size and different in shape. Central to the geniculate, the field defects of the two eyes become more congruous, that is, more similar in shape and size. Large interruptions of the visual pathway in the optic radiations of one cortex, or affecting the occipital cortex itself, produce a homonymous hemianopia (Figure 23.2). Even an extensive or complete loss of one half of each visual field is sometimes unnoticed by the patient.

The optic discs and related fundus appearances
Three factors need to be considered when the optic discs are being examined:

1 Pallor of the discs, referred to as optic atrophy

2 Swelling of the discs

3 Ophthalmic signs associated with pallor and oedema of the discs.

Disc pallor—optic atrophy

If the optic disc is obviously pale, the pallor may be general (global), or more marked on the temporal side (temporal). Although temporal pallor is traditionally the type of atrophy encountered in demyelination, it is likely that many cases of progressive atrophy initially proceed through a stage of temporal pallor (Figures 23.3 and 23.4).

A comparison should be made between the optic disc of the two eyes if there is any doubt as to the appearance of one of them. The association of disc pallor with some defect of the visual field, or even of the vision itself, is very significant. There is no direct correlation between the degree of disc pallor and visual function because the pallor is due, at least partially, to diminution of the blood supply to the disc.

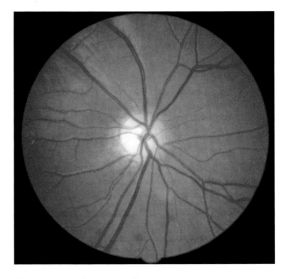

Figure 23.3   Optic atrophy.

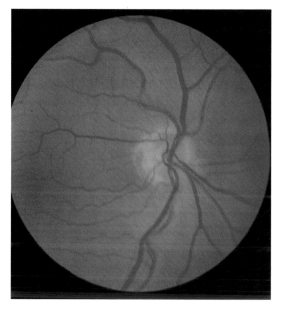

a

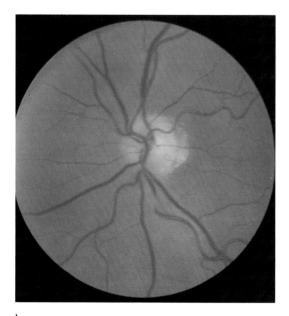

b

Figure 23.4 Temporal pallor of the left optic disc (*b*). Compare with the normal right disc (*a*).

In discussing glaucoma (see Chapter 13), it was noted that sometimes a central cup is present in a normal optic disc and the floor of the disc is often pale. In assessing an optic disc for pathological degrees of pallor, where a cup is present, the part of the disc surrounding the cup deserves special attention. These cups are sometimes quite large (especially in myopes) and may give a false impression of atrophy. Nevertheless, simple glaucoma is the most common condition producing optic atrophy.

Optic atrophy arises from disorders of the fibres of the optic nerve itself, or of the ganglion cells giving rise to these fibres. A disorder of the ganglion cells is referred to as 'primary' optic atrophy because it occurs, for example, in tertiary syphilis. Conditions affecting the fibres include those due to compression by space occupying lesions, either intraorbital or intracranial; these cases are called 'secondary' optic atrophy.

In a third group, as outlined below, the condition is the end-result of processes that start with disc swelling.

Swollen optic discs

The normal optic disc has sharply defined edges. Where the definition of the edges is doubtful, or they are blurred, there are several possible causes. For example, some normal optic discs have blurred or slightly swollen edges, and are small overall, due to crowding of the nerve fibres. The condition is called pseudo papilloedema and usually occurs in hypermetropes (Figure 23.5). A marked refractive error (severe astigmatism, for example) may make focusing clearly on the disc margins impossible. In other cases, abnormal white deposits deep in the substance of the disc margins (drusen) may pile up and blur the edges of the disc (Figure 23.6a). Another cause of indefinite disc margins is opaque retinal nerve fibres (Figure 23.6b).

The most important clinical cause of blurring of the disc margins is oedema, that is, accumulation of fluid in the nerve head leading to the swollen disc.

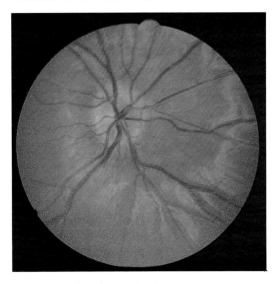

Figure 23.5   Pseudo papilloedema.

The swollen disc with normal vision

The appearance of an obviously swollen optic disc in a patient with no particular visual disturbance or loss of vision is referred to as papilloedema. A fully developed example of this condition is easy to recognize (Figure 23.7):

● The disc is red and engorged with elevated edges

● The retinal veins are significantly dilated and tortuous and there may also be haemorrhage alongside them

● The condition is often bilateral and one disc may be more swollen than the other.

There may be no ocular or visual symptoms until the condition is advanced and of long standing.

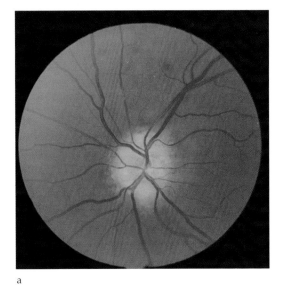

a

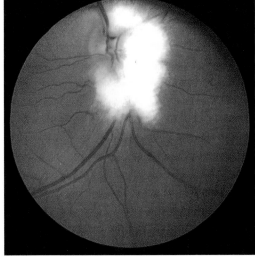

b

Figure 23.6   (*a*) Drusen of the optic disc. (*b*) Opaque nerve fibres.

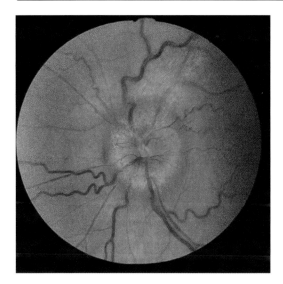

Figure 23.7   Papilloedema.

For example, a disc of doubtful appearance, which is in fact due to a very early papilloedema, has many fine vessels on and within it that leak fluorescein. This persists for some time in the disc and the surrounding retina.

The cause of the swelling is not known for certain, but there seem to be two important elements: fluid leakage from small vessels, and swelling of the nerve fibres themselves owing to obstructed axoplasmic flow. Both of these factors are believed to be precipitated by the elevation of the cerebrospinal fluid pressure in the sheath surrounding the optic nerves, affecting the fibres directly or compressing the central retinal vein as it emerges from the optic nerve.

The most important cause of papilloedema is therefore raised intracranial pressure. In most cases a well defined cause such as a space-occupying lesion is found, but there are a number of cases where no particular aetiological factor is identified. One of these is known as 'benign intracranial hypertension', which appears to be a specific clinical entity comprising headache, marked papilloedema and occasionally with a VIth nerve palsy.

Another important cause of papilloedema is high blood pressure, which may occur with only slight hypertensive changes in the rest of the retina; more usually, though, it is part of a very florid hypertensive fundus picture (see page 220).

CT scanning is always performed in cases of papilloedema suspected to be due to raised intracranial pressure.

Ultimately, however, optic atrophy will supervene, with the disc becoming pale. At that stage, progressive failure of vision will occur. Even at an earlier stage, a transient momentary loss of vision is sometimes a feature, although the sight is generally very good. (An enlargement of the blind spot may be found on testing the central field, although this is a suggestive and not a conclusive sign.)

The recognition of an early papilloedema is partly a matter of experience and partly a matter of investigation, although certain diagnosis can be difficult. The swelling itself is believed to start on the nasal edge of the disc, with the temporal edges being left relatively clearly defined. Should a cup be present, it is usually filled at an early stage and it is said that the preservation of the cup, and the presence of venous pulsation, are factors against the diagnosis of papilloedema.

In some circumstances, fluorescein retinal angiography has proved helpful in diagnosis.

The swollen disc with loss of vision

Whereas papilloedema appears to be largely a passive hydrodynamic response, there are conditions where fluid accumulation at the disc is an active result of some different pathological process, perhaps inflammatory or ischaemic. In this case, there is some loss of visual function; the type and extent of the loss depends on the nature of the condition. The two most important clinical pictures are acute optic neuritis (presenting as 'papillitis') and ischaemic papillopathy (Figures 23.8 and 23.9).

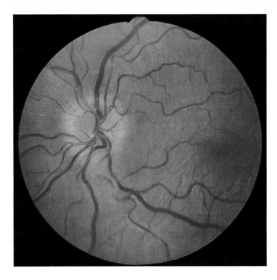

Figure 23.8 Optic neuritis.

The swollen disc with loss of vision is likely to present acutely, the loss of vision often being marked and the condition usually unilateral. The disc swelling itself may not be severe and any venous congestion is confined to the immediate vicinity of the disc. Associated with the loss of vision, pupillary phenomena are often disturbed.

Because of these special characteristics, there should not be any difficulty in differentiating papilloedema from papillitis (see page 232). Occasionally, however, inflammatory swelling of the disc may result from a general intraocular inflammation such as a low-grade uveitis. It may also be noted in cases of retinal vasculitis, although this is a rather ill-defined diagnostic category.

When both eyes are involved and the vision is slightly, if at all, affected, such cases may resemble the picture of raised intracranial pressure. It is therefore important in any case of a swelling of the optic disc to be sure of the presence or absence of inflammatory disease in the eye. Indeed, it may be that oedema of the retina spreading on to the disc will cause the appearance of papilloedema.

Disc swelling associated with acute loss of vision will usually subside in a matter of weeks and the optic disc will then simply show pallor.

Related fundus appearances

Pale optic discs result from any widespread ocular or retinal disease associated with death of the ganglion cells. Indeed, we have noted the commonest cause of optic atrophy is chronic simple glaucoma, but here the cupping of the disc, and the finding of a raised intraocular pressure, make the diagnosis and differentiate it from other causes (see page 113).

Major vascular occlusions, retinal degeneration of the retinitis pigmentosa type, even an extensive senile macular degeneration, may all be accompanied by pale discs. The point is that in these instances the pallor of the disc is not the main abnormal fundus finding. In fact

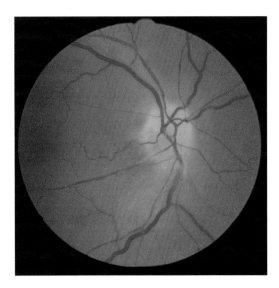

Figure 23.9 Ischaemic papillopathy.

these cases are referred to as 'consecutive optic atrophy'.

Ocular movements   Chapter 19 emphasized the distinction between the two fundamental varieties of strabismus: the concomitant type arising in childhood and the paralytic squint which may arise at any time in life. The latter is the form with which the neurologist is most likely to be concerned.

Weakness of paralysis of one or other extensive ocular muscle may arise from some abnormality of its nerve supply or because the muscle itself is in some way abnormal (neurogenic or myogenic weakness, for example). The main symptom is diplopia (double vision).

In the common neurogenic type of paralysis, typical patterns develop according to the nerves (IIIrd, IVth or VIth) affected. Diplopia is experienced when the eyes move in the direction of action of the affected muscle, or muscles. Indeed, clinically it is often possible to identify the paresed muscle by having the patient follow with the eyes alone, keeping the head still, a small torch bulb and then to state when the separation of the two images is the greatest. One eye is then covered to identify from which the farthest displaced image is arising; because of the inversion of retinal images, this eye is the one with the paresed muscle or muscles.

In a VIth or abducens nerve palsy, the affected eye is usually slightly convergent when the individual is looking straight ahead and it cannot be moved fully outwards in the direction of the paralysed lateral rectus; in this direction, diplopia is experienced with horizontal separation of the images (Figure 23.10).

A IVth or trochlear nerve palsy is uncommon; but because the IVth nerve is the sole supply to the superior oblique muscle, diplopia is experienced with a vertically separated image and is particularly marked when the individual looks down to the opposite side.

In a IIIrd or oculomotor nerve palsy, the eye is usually slightly divergent; adduction, elevation and depression are all limited, with only abduction being unaffected (Figure 23.11). In addition,

as part of a IIIrd nerve palsy there may be ptosis and dilatation of the pupil if the fibres supplying the voluntary part of the levator and the parasympathetic supply to the pupil sphincter have been affected. The ptosis may be so marked that it prevents double vision. Ischaemic lesions of the nerve nucleus are unlikely to involve the pupil.

The ptosis of a IIIrd nerve palsy should be easily distinguished from that in Horner's syndrome of sympathetic paralysis (see Figure 16.7), the latter being characterized by a relatively small pupil. The other two components of this syndrome are enophthalmos (recession of the eye, which may simply be a false appearance) and anhidrosis (failure of sweating so that the affected side of the face may feel warmer than the normal side). There is of course no defect of ocular movement.

Gaze palsies   Homonymous field defects occurring in major strokes may also be associated with gaze palsies. The eyes remain parallel, but are often deviated (conjugate deviation) away from the paralysed side of the body and cannot be moved to that side.

Nystagmus   The other important sign which may be seen on examination of the ocular movements is nystagmus, an oscillatory or jerky movement of the eyes due to a failure to maintain fixation. This is a very complex subject and one to which a whole book could be devoted. In appropriate circumstances, nystagmus is a physiological response to movement in the outside world. This 'optokinetic' or physiological nystagmus (see page 250) occurs in a subject looking at a passing scene where a sequence of fixation, loss of fixation and refixation repeats itself.

Pathological nystagmus can be divided as follows:

- Congenital nystagmus (early infantile)

- Acquired nystagmus.

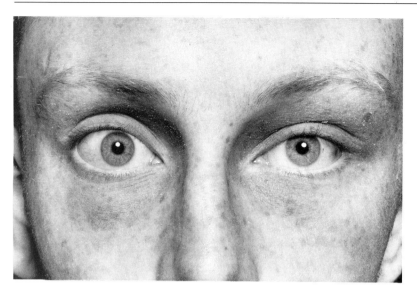

a

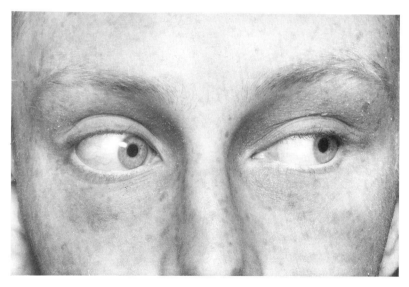

b

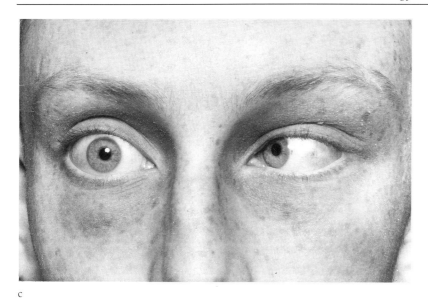

c

Figure 23.10 Ocular movements in a case of right abducens nerve palsy: (*a*) shows the straight ahead appearance. On looking to the left the eyes are straight. On looking to the right a convergent strabismus is present as the right eye cannot move outwards.

Congenital nystagmus (early infantile) is often described as being a pendular or jelly-like or wobbly movement. The oscillations are most commonly horizontal, but are sometimes vertical. In virtually all cases of congenital nystagmus, and incidentally in the great majority of acquired nystagmus, patients do not have any sensation of the movement of the external world.

Congenital nystagmus is often present in all positions of the gaze, although it may be more marked in one particular direction, and a compensatory head posture may be adopted so that the oscillations are least marked. The associated history is very important. In many cases, congenital nystagmus is known to have been present since early life, and often goes with

defective vision either as the cause or effect. There may be macular lesions, congenital cataract or albinism, partial or fully developed. Nystagmus can also occur when the fundi are visible and normal. In some cases, there is a family history of the condition.

Latent nystagmus is an interesting variant of the congenital type. Here the oscillatory movements are much more marked if one or other eye is covered; in fact, they may be hardly noticeable with neither eye covered. Along with this, it has been found that the vision of either eye tested separately with the other covered is much worse than that of the two eyes together, the binocular

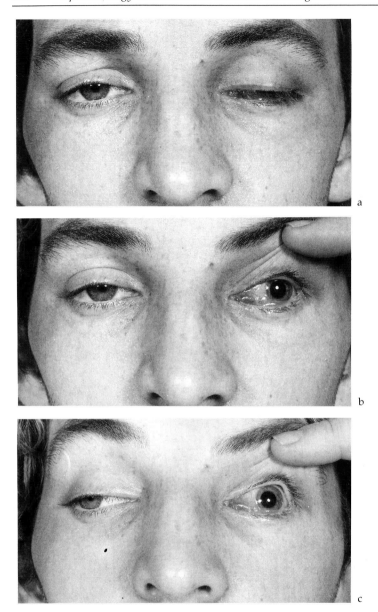

Figure 23.11 Ocular movements in a case of left oculomotor nerve palsy: (*a*) and (*b*) show the position of the eyes looking straight ahead. There is left ptosis and on raising the upper lid the left eye can be seen to be divergent. (*c*) shows that on right gaze the left eye does not adduct at all. In (*d*) the left eye is shown to abduct normally on left gaze. (*e*) and (*f*) indicate that elevation and depression of the affected left eye are grossly impaired. The left pupil is dilated and fixed.

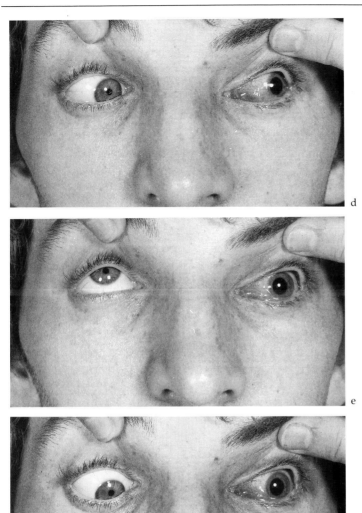

d

e

f

visual acuity. In a normal subject, the vision of the two eyes used together is slightly better than of the two used separately; in latent nystagmus the superiority of the binocular visual acuity is considerable.

Acquired nystagmus is often described as being jerky, with a fast and slow phase. It is the direction of the fast phase that characterizes nystagmus, even though the slow phase is the pathological element, the fast one being merely a refixation. The movements are commonly horizontal, with or without a rotary element. Vertical nystagmus is much less common.

Broadly, this 'jerky' nystagmus is of fairly sudden onset in adults, and indicates involvement of the lower brain stem or of the VIIIth nerve labyrinthine mechanism. Its occurrence in a patient complaining of dizziness is therefore of some significance. Some particular varieties of acqured nystagmus are discussed in Chapter 24.

The pupil From a neurological standpoint, examination of the pupils' size and reactions, and the similarity of each to its fellow is of major concern. It is as well to remember that the pupil is the hole in the iris and that the iris is part of the eye. An abnormality of the size or reaction of the pupil may be the result of an existing or previous ocular disease, hence the importance of examining the pupil when an acute red eye is present (see Chapter 3).

The size of the pupils

Although in most normal subjects the pupils are of equal size, inequality (anisocoria), if not marked and if unaccompanied by any abnormality of the pupillary reflexes, is often of no importance, and may be congenital. Occasionally it does indicate some neurological disturbance such as Horner's syndrome (see page 235), or an oculomotor nerve malfunction. Note should therefore be made of any associated ptosis or defect of ocular movement.

Loss of pupil reactions

Normally the pupil constricts in response to light, the iris acting as the shutter of the optical system to prevent damage to the retina. Constriction of the pupil also occurs on accommodation and associated convergence for near vision; this may give some optical benefit.

The reactions, both to light and to accommodation, are reflexes which involve an afferent limb, a central pathway and an efferent limb.

1 The efferent limb is via the parasympathetic to the pupil sphincter for both reactions

2 The afferent limb of the light reflex is via fibres from the retina, predominantly the central retina, which bypass the lateral geniculate body and enter the upper midbrain

3 The afferent stimulus to the accommodation reflex is more complex, probably involving higher cortical functions.

The pupils' reactions are normally bilateral and light shone on either eye causes both pupils to constrict.

In order to describe the abnormalities of pupil function, we should recognize and define the terms 'direct' and 'consensual' reaction.

● Direct reaction to light is the response of the pupil of the eye on to which the light is shone

● The consensual response is the reaction of the pupil to light shone on the other eye.

In a motor paralysis of one pupil, the reaction to light of that pupil is diminshed both directly and consensually. Reaction to light of the pupil on the other side is normal both directly and consensually.

In a sensory paralysis of one pupil, the direct reaction of that pupil and the consensual reaction of the other pupil are both diminished or lost. Consensual reaction of the pupil on the affected side and the direct light reaction of the other pupil are both normal. This afferent defect is seen at its most typical in a blind eye. Unreacting dilated pupils occur when both eyes are blind, and are also an important sign of death.

Combinations of altered size and reactions

These are commonly found where a relatively large pupil has poor or absent reactions to light or accommodation, or both. The possibility of an ocular cause should always be considered. Traumatic mydriasis (see page 176), past herpes zoster, local intended or inadvertent atropiniz-ation, even past or existing closed angle glaucoma, should all be considered first before a neurological cause is sought.

A particular oddity is Adie's syndrome, or myotonic pupil, where a very marked slowing of the light reaction (direct and consensual) of usually just one pupil occurs. It is commonly found in the young and in females. The pupil tends to be relatively dilated and even the accommodation convergence reaction is often impaired, although on prolonged near gaze a slow decrease in size develops. Adie's syndrome is occasionally associated with the loss of one or other of the deep reflexes, knee jerk or ankle jerk, but there are no other neurological signs. The pupillary dilatation may occasionally be accompanied by blurred near vision due to an associated interference with accommodation. If this symptom or photophobia are marked, weak miotic drops such as 0.5 per cent pilocarpine may be helpful.

Loss of light reaction traditionally brings to mind the Argyll Robertson pupil of tertiary syphilis. When this picture is classically present, complete loss of light reaction of both pupils is found. This occurs in combination with an exaggerated fast contraction on accommodation, even though initially the pupils in this condition are bilaterally very small. Nowadays the con-dition is extremely rare and there should be no difficulty in differentiating it from other ins-tances of loss of light reaction.

The commonest cause of bilateral small pupils, with loss of all reactions, is of course the miosis produced in cases of glaucoma through the use of miotic drops, usually pilocarpine (see Chapter

13). Other causes include opiate toxicity and brain stem, particularly mid-brain, injuries.

An important abnormal pupil reaction occurs in cases of defective central vision in one eye. The pupil, although not necessarily abnormally large, has an ill-sustained constriction to light shone directly on the eye. When this direct light follows the transfer of light from the other eye, the pupil of the affected eye dilates slightly. This is because the consensual dilatation induced by withdrawing light from the normal eye is more powerful than the direct constricting effect of light on the affected eye.

This 'afferent pupil defect', shown by what is sometimes called the swinging light test, is thought by some neurologists to be solely charac-teristic of the central visual loss of acute optic neuritis; as can be seen in this chapter, that is not so, although it is certainly a valuable aid in the diagnosis of the condition.

Proptosis and enophthalmos Proptosis and enophthalmos may give a clue to the orbital pathology, some of which may arise intra-cranially. Even though proptosis and enophthal-mos themselves are not common neurologically, they can be of great importance if other abnorma-lities such as disturbance of the ocular movement or pupil are present.

The position and function of the eyelids This has been dealt with in Chapter 17 and, from a neurological standpoint, the important findings are lagophthalmos (VIIth nerve dysfunction) and ptosis (IIIrd nerve or sympathetic disorder).

Facial weakness is of general diagnostic importance; but it can also have serious ocular implications, particularly if the cornea is incom-pletely covered.

The corneal sensitivity Corneal numbness points to the sensory root of the trigeminal nerve. For example, it is an important sign of an acoustic neuroma, the characteristic tumour of the cerebello-pontine angle. It is worth remem-bering that corneal anaesthesia may have ocular causes (see Chapter 8). The herpes viruses of both varieties may cause a keratitis and lead to loss of corneal sensitivity. Reduced sensitivity is also a consequence of prolonged contact lens wear.

Any neurological condition affecting the brain stem and producing corneal numbness and facial weakness is particularly hazardous for the cornea (see page 162), which is both insensitive and unprotected.

PRACTICAL POINTS

● The cranial nerves II to VIII and the autonomic system are all involved in a routine neuro-ophthalmic examination.

● Field defects are among the commonest visual neurological disorders. Both field defects and central visual loss are important signs of neurological disease where no other symptoms are present.

● 'Primary' optic atrophy arises from disorders of the fibres of the optic nerve itself, or its ganglion cells. 'Secondary' optic atrophy is due to compression by space-occupying lesions.

● A swollen optic disc appears blurred at the edges, a condition known as papilloedema. The most important cause is raised intracranial pressure. Ultimately, optic atrophy and progressive failure of vision may result.

● Eye movements are affected in neurological disease according to the nerves involved, often leading to strabismus and diplopia. Other associated conditions are ptosis and alteration of pupil size.

● Proptosis and enophthalmos, while not normally neurological, may be significant in this context. They may be associated with disturbance of ocular movement.

Major neuro-ophthalmological diseases

The major neuro-ophthalmological disorders are considered under the following categories:

- Cerebral vascular disease
- Intracranial space-occupying lesions
- Demyelination
- Functional loss of vision
- Myasthenia gravis
- Orbital disease.

Cerebral vascular disease

A substantial part of neurology is concerned with disease of the blood supply to the head and brain. Three groups of the conditions are of particular importance in relation to ophthalmology:

1 Major intracerebral vessel disorders

2 Aneurysms of the circle of Willis

3 Cranial arteritis.

Major intracerebral vessel disorders (strokes)

Serious disturbances of the cerebral blood flow have particular ophthalmological effects, and we have already noted that similar temporary phenomena may result from spasm of the cerebral vessels in hypertensive encephalopathy.

Longer lasting effects on the vision result from strokes caused by cerebral infarction, by embolism or thrombosis, the last occurring in a vessel showing arteriosclerosis or hypertensive changes, or both. These may involve the optic radiations, the suprageniculate part of the visual pathway (which is that between the lateral geniculate body and the occipital cortex), or the visual cortex itself. Any disturbances at these sites will produce homonymous defects, with loss of all or part of the half-field of each eye. The most extensive lesions lead to a complete loss of these half-fields — homonymous hemianopia (see page 229).

Certainly a patient suffering a major stroke, often from disturbance of the middle cerebral artery or its branches, leading to any kind of unilateral motor or sensory loss, should be suspected of having homonymous field loss. It is, however, not uncommon for a patient to present with an isolated homonymous defect without any other neurological signs.

Curiously enough, visual field loss may not be recognized by patients until it is pointed out to them, although they frequently realize there is something wrong but cannot formulate it. The visual disability is often ascribed to one particular eye, the patient failing to realize that it is the fields of both eyes that are affected.

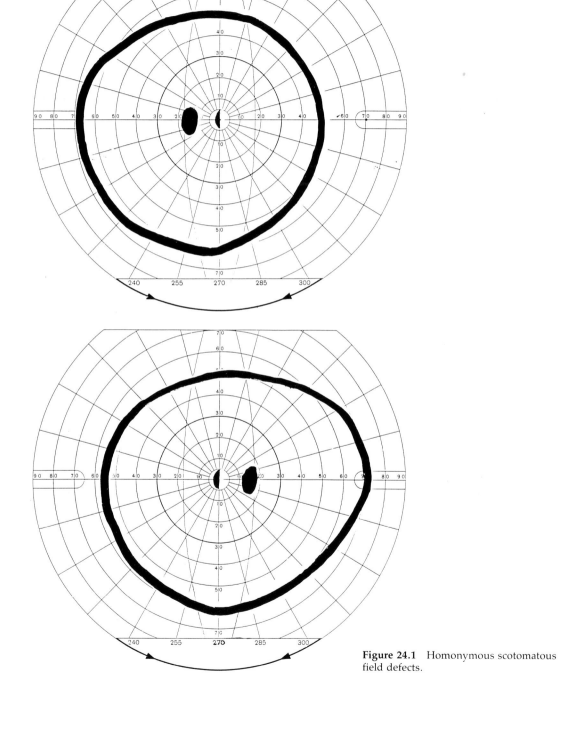

Figure 24.1 Homonymous scotomatous field defects.

A common complaint is difficulty with reading left to right. The next word is not seen in a right homonymous defect, or the beginning of the next line is hard to find in a left homonymous defect.

If parts of the radiation or visual cortex on one side remain unaffected, quadrantic or scotomatous homonymous defects result which are usually fairly congruous (Figure 24.1). In accordance with the general principle that, once destroyed, central nervous neurones do not regenerate, field defects produced by stroke are largely permanent and no treatment is available.

Whatever the extent of suprageniculate lesions, they hardly ever produce a vertical split in central vision, which would be very much noticed by the patient. This phenomenon of macular sparing may stem from the fact that the macular area of the retina is bilaterally represented in the cortex and because each occipital cortical tip (the site of macular representation) has a blood supply from both the middle and posterior cerebral arteries. The macula may be spared, even if there is bilateral occipital lobe infarction. This is so-called 'cortical blindness' and typically develops when an already hemianopic patient develops a hemianopia on the other side. It is one example of 'tunnel vision' (extremely small visual fields) (Figure 24.2), of which the other common organic causes are advanced bilateral chronic simple glaucoma and late stage retinitis pigmentosa. Temporary tunnel vision may occur in migraine and it may also be a hysterical phenomenon.

Significant cerebral haemorrhage is usually fatal, but in the period of unconsciousness preceding death, conjugate deviation of the eyes may be noted.

Vertebro-basilar insufficiency, besides affecting the posterior cerebral arteries, and therefore the visual cortex, may also cause brain stem signs which may include involvement of the oculomotor nuclei with paresis or paralysis of one or more extraocular muscles or their interconnections, leading to diplopia or nystagmus, or both.

Embolic cerebral disease may occur along with embolic retinal disease, whether the source of the emboli is cardiac or in the carotid circulation. Commonly, the patient's history reveals transient attacks of loss of vision in one eye that may finally lead to a major retinal arterial obstruction and blindness, perhaps followed by a major stroke with a contralateral hemiplegia.

During and for a short period after such attacks of transient loss of vision (TIAs, 'amaurosis fugax'), the retinal vessels may show emboli either of cholesterol plaques or of platelets. Early recognition of the condition prompts medical or surgical treatment for the source of the emboli, usually in the ipsilateral internal carotid artery, and may prevent a major stroke occurring. Clinical ausculation and carotid angiography, both conventional and digital subtraction, are carried out where appropriate.

It must be admitted, however, that the majority of subjects giving a history of transient visual loss show no abnormal clinical findings and investigation reveals no source of emboli or any general vascular disease. There is often but not always a history of true migraine, and certainly in younger subjects such episodes are likely to be 'migraine without headache', also known as 'migraine equivalents'.

Aneurysms of the circle of Willis

There are several different ways in which an aneurysm may impinge upon ophthalmology:

1 As a space-occupying lesion leading to compression of the lower visual pathways (see below)

2 Sudden enlargement may occur, leading to interference with neighbouring nerves, particularly the oculomotor, and the ophthalmic division of the trigeminal. Pain in the region of the eye, perhaps with diplopia, dulling of corneal sensation and a dilated pupil may be found. The clinical picture is sometimes referred to as ophthalmoplegic migraine.

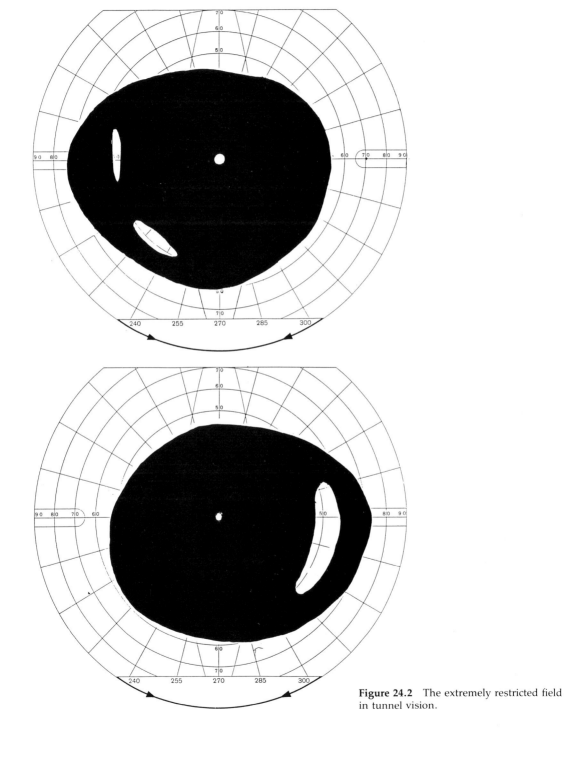

Figure 24.2   The extremely restricted field in tunnel vision.

3 By rupture, leading to a subarachnoid haemorrhage. The eyes may show retinal haemorrhages, occasionally large and sub-hyaloid (between the retina and vitreous) in situation. These can burst forward to give vitreous haemorrhage, leading to a serious sudden loss of vision. How these haemorrhages arise is not clear, though possibly they are caused by blood in the cerebral spinal fluid entering the eye along the optic nerve sheath. Alternatively, the retinal venous drainage may be embarrassed by the cerebral spinal fluid pressure as the central vein emerges from the optic nerve across the subarachnoid space.

Cranial arteritis

The condition is also known as 'temporal arteritis' or 'giant cell arteritis' and is rarely seen in patients under the age of sixty-five years. The arteritis is widespread and may initially affect vessels remote from the eyes or head. In such cases, months of general malaise are followed by sudden severe headache. On examination the superficial temporal artery is non-pulsatile, inflamed and tender. Other clinical features include fever, weight loss and pain on chewing. A biopsy of the artery shows an inflammatory condition characterized by the presence of giant cells. The aetiology is unknown, but it is believed to be related to the other collagen diseases such as polyarteritis nodosa and systemic lupus erythematosus, as well as the milder condition of polymyalgia rheumatica.

The important eye condition associated with cranial arteritis is ischaemic papillopathy, which is due to the involvement of the small vessels supplying the tissues of the optic nerve head. This circulation is independent of the retinal circulation, but it is so vital in the conduction and function of the optic nerve that, if it is interfered with, complete blindness results, usually very suddenly. In such an eye the fundus signs are minimal, the disc being slightly swollen, often with a pale centre. The retinal circulation is normal, thus distinguishing it from a retinal artery occlusion. The pupil fails to react to light.

If one eye is affected by cranial arteritis, the fellow eye may also become affected very quickly. It is therefore vital to confirm the diagnosis by an emergency estimation of the ESR (erythrocyte sedimentation rate), which is always raised and often very high indeed; for example, in the region of 100 mmHg per hour. If appropriate, a temporal artery biopsy should be undertaken, but it is not essential. A negative histology should not be regarded as excluding the condition, as cranial arteritis is notoriously patchy in the vessels it affects.

High doses of systemic steroids (60–80 mg of prednisolone per day) should be given once the blood has been tested and these should be adjusted according to the lowering of the ESR The vision of the affected eye unfortunately rarely returns, but the fellow eye is saved by this routine.

Cranial arteritis may affect other parts of the central nervous system and the ophthalmologist sometimes encounters hemianopias and oculomotor palsies from this cause.

The picture of sudden loss of vision due to ischaemic papillopathy is sometimes seen in patients who do not appear to have cranial arteritis. It is assumed that the interference in the circulation of the nerve head is simply arteriosclerotic.

Intracranial space-occupying lesions

The traditional description of intracranial space-occupying lesions divides them into those external to the brain substance and those within it. In ophthalmology, this subdivision is recognized as:

- Lower visual pathway compression
- Intracerebral lesions.

Lower visual pathway compression

The lower visual pathways may be compressed by numerous lesions. The three most common are:

1 Meningioma

2 Basal aneurysm

3 Pituitary-related swelling, either intrasellar of endocrine origin, or suprasellar (cranio-pharyngioma).

The ophthalmological presentation may be blindness, in some cases quite sudden, or poor vision in one eye if the condition is predominantly of one optic nerve, or it may be a bitemporal hemianopia with a degree of symmetry that varies between cases if there is significant chiasmal compression (see Figure 23.1). Tract pressure is uncommon. Optic atrophy on one or both sides may be obvious, but it is worth noting that defective vision can be present for considerable periods before pallor or atrophy of the optic disc is found. Field defects should always be looked for, especially to red objects, whatever the appearance of the disc.

    If lower visual pathway compression is suspected, either from the visual history or from ancillary symptoms and signs, whether headache, endocrine changes (acromegaly, for example), pupillary or oculomotor anomalies, full investigation is mandatory. Simple radiography, CT scanning and arteriography are called for and, where indicated, a neurosurgical opinion should be sought at an early date.

Intracerebral lesions

Involvement of the optic radiations and visual cortex by gliomata or secondary deposits produces corresponding defects of the visual fields. Such lesions, particularly gliomata, may cause raised intracranial pressure and are always the clinician's first suspicion in a patient presenting with severe headache who shows bilateral papilloedema.

    Infiltration by the tumour of the visual pathways in the cortex may produce sensations of flashes of light, but this is rare.

    Brain stem tumours may involve the oculomotor nerves, producing diplopia, and their involvement provides valuable localizing signs.

Interference with cerebrospinal fluid circulation may lead to papilloedema.

Demyelination

In its major disease, multiple sclerosis, demyelination may produce a whole host of ophthalmic symptoms and signs. There are, however, some clinical pictures in ophthalmology that are thought to be fairly typical of the condition:

● Acute optic neuritis

● Ocular muscle involvement

● Miscellaneous signs.

Acute optic neuritis

Although the '-itis' implies an inflammatory aetiology, this is recognized as a misnomer. However it is accepted that, associated with an acute patch of demyelination, there may be evidence of an inflammation. Should such a patch of demyelination affect the optic nerve, it particularly involves the papillomacular bundle and produces sudden loss of vision, with a central scotoma. Optic neuritis presents in two forms:

1 **Papillitis** A change in the appearance of the optic disc will be present if the demyelinated patch is close to the end of the optic nerve (these signs are described on page 233).

2 **Retrobulbar neuritis** This is said to occur where the patch of demyelination in the optic nerve is farther away from the eye; there are no fundus signs.

In retrobulbar neuritis, the clinical problem appears to be that of an eye with a normal fundus and poorly corrected visual acuity (see page 249).

    In acute neuritis of either variety, papillitis or retrobulbar neuritis, there are associated signs, some of which seem to indicate an inflammation. There is pain, particularly on moving the eye, and the eye may be tender to touch at the end of the superior rectus insertion. Most significant is the sensory loss of the pupil shown by the swinging light test (see page 241).

In a typical case, the vision may be less than 6/60, the top letter on the Snellen chart (see page 32). An obvious central scotoma is present even in a confrontation comparative field test. Such a finding is virtually never encountered in a functional loss of vision and confirms the diagnosis. The latency of the visually evoked response (VER) should be investigated.

The VER is an electroencephalographic (EEG) recording of the visual cortex in response to a rhythmic stimulus to the eye, such as an alternating chequerboard pattern. Computer analysis of the resulting EEG sorts out what the relevant local response is amid the general brain activity. The important measurement is the delay in eye-to-cortex time. Normally this is about 100 milliseconds, and this is typically prolonged in optic neuritis. The amplitude of the visual evoked response may be related to the visual acuity.

Signs of demyelination may be found elsewhere, or there may be a history of confirmed or suggestive episodes. Acute optic neuritis is, however, frequently the first episode of multiple sclerosis. The development of other features may be delayed or never occur. This last fact has prompted suggestions of causes other than demyelination for the condition as, for example, inflammation of nearby structures such as paranasal sinuses.

If treatment is to be given for acute optic neuritis, a course of systemic steroids is suggested. It is debatable, however, whether this will make any difference as most cases recover completely in about six to eight weeks. The optic disc, whether previously involved or not, slowly develops temporal pallor. A small proportion do not recover at all, the central visual loss being permanent and the disc becoming very pale indeed.

Ocular muscle involvement

A fleeting involvement of the extraocular muscles may produce diplopia in which the precise muscle involved is difficult to identify. There is a curious picture said to be characteristic of demyelination. This is internuclear ophthalmoplegia, which may be due to involvement of the medial longitudinal bundle in the brain stem connecting the nuclei of the oculomotor and trochlear nuclei in the mid-brain with the abducens nucleus in the pons; demyelination seems to have a particular predilection for it. In internuclear ophthalmolplegia, adduction of each eye is absent on lateral gaze to either side, but convergence is normal, showing that both medial recti are still able to respond.

Associated with the condition is ataxic nystagmus in which on lateral movement the amplitude of the jerks of the abducting eye is very great, the adducting eye jerking slightly, if at all.

Miscellaneous ophthalmic signs in demyelination

In longstanding multiple sclerosis, severe eye involvement is not uncommon. Progressive loss of vision, leading to blindness due to chronic demyelination of the optic nerve, often occurs. Marked nystagmus and manifest paralytic squint may be present and a variety of pupillary anomalies are encountered.

Functional loss of vision

One of the most important and difficult problems in clinical ophthalmology is to decide the cause of poor sight when in the presence of a normal fundus, vision is defective even with the appropriate spectacle correction.

In all cases of defective vision of this type, it is important to pay particular attention to the pupil's reaction for signs of an afferent defect (see page 241), and it is essential to examine the central visual field of both eyes for a central scotoma.

A full neurological investigation may be indicated as there may be some involvement of the visual pathway (perhaps the optic nerve itself), in which the changes have not yet manifested themselves as a pale disc.

Among the non-neurological conditions which might produce this picture are amblyopia, hysteria and malingering.

Amblyopia

The condition is due either to a high, long-standing refractive error in one eye (anisometropia), or associated with childhood squint. It is discussed in more detail on page 185).

Hysteria

The suspicion of hysterical loss of vision may arise from the general demeanour of the patient. For example, the patient often shows a remarkable ability to avoid circumstances of potential injury. Bizarre visual field changes such as spiralling are sometimes present.

Malingering

Malingering is found in medico-legal cases involving compensation and in those persons trying to avoid unpleasant obligations such as military service. A form of malingering is occasionally seen in schoolchildren, usually in the eight- to twelve-year-old age group where the precipitating factor may be jealousy of a classmate who has recently acquired spectacles, or through some anxiety about an approaching educational hurdle. An introspective attention to the eyes develops with complaints of blurred vision, attacks of blindness, headaches and so on.

Tests to identify malingering depend on being able to trick the patient in some way. A typical method to use in a patient with functional loss of vision in one eye is to ask for the Snellen chart to be read with both eyes open, with a powerful blurring lens placed in front of the normal eye. Children often read down the chart amazingly

well through lenses put in a trial frame with the equivalent power being nil, presumably being encouraged by the general panoply of the equipment and the prospect of needing spectacles.

Among more recherché tests for malingering is the induction of optokinetic nystagmus. A drum with black and white stripes is rotated in front of the patient. No one with normal visual apparatus can resist the oscillatory motion of the eyes produced by the rotation. In fact, from the width of the stripes and the rotation speed, it is possible to gauge the patient's visual acuity. Electrophysiological investigations (ERG and EOG, q.v.) are also sometimes helpful.

It should be mentioned again that the suspicion as to a functional visual loss may be aroused by the gross nature of the complaint in the presence of brisk pupil reactions.

Malingering has to be finely judged. The decision to diagnose such cases always raises the question of whether or not to embark on extensive investigations of an apparently 'inexplicable' visual defect with a possibility of reinforcing some functional factor and increasing the general anxiety about the problem. In many cases, it is wise to temporize and observe the patient over a period of say two or three months, during which time such a functional factor may disappear and the situation resolve itself.

Myasthenia gravis

The ophthalmologist is often involved in this failure of neuromuscular transmission, which is believed to be an autoimmune disorder of the motor end plate, characterized by a blocking of the post-synaptic membrane by an anti-acetylcholine receptor antibody.

Notoriously variable in its early stages, myasthenia gravis may show itself as a recurrent ptosis or as diplopia. The history of an inability to keep the eyes open late in the day, perhaps associated with some difficulty in swallowing or chewing, should alert the practitioner to the possibility of the condition. It is one that the ophthalmologist tends to miss as very often the signs of any abnormality are absent at the time of the examination. Intentionally fatiguing the levator by repeated blinking may cause a ptosis. In any doubtful case, referral to a neurologist for a tensilon test is essential.

The established case requires lifelong treatment with parasympathomimetic therapy (prostigmine or similar). Thymectomy is helpful in selective cases. Immunosuppression is now playing an important role in treatment.

Myasthenia, although usually a generalized condition affecting functions such as swallowing and breathing, is sometimes limited to the eye muscles (ocular myasthenia).

Other myopathic disorders may also affect the eye muscles, causing ptosis and diplopia. The association of myotonic dystrophy with cataract has already been noted in Chapter 10.

Orbital disease

Orbital pathology may have important neurological associations. An infiltrative or space-occupying lesion of the orbit itself, or near to one of the orbital fissures, may involve the optic nerve as well as the structures entering the apex of the orbit—the IIIrd, IVth, Vth and VIth nerves. The proptosis that results may mechanically interfere with the action of the extrinsic ocular muscles.

The commonest condition affecting the orbit in this way is dysthyroid infiltration (see Chapter 25), but specific granulomatous involvement known as pseudo-tumour, lacrimal gland tumours, congenital vessel anomalies such as cavernous hemiangioma and mucocoeles or tumours of the surrounding sinuses are all encountered. CT scanning, and to some extent ultrasound, are valuable aids in the differential diagnosis of orbital lesions. Accuracy of diagnosis allows for a rational and appropriate therapeutic approach—whether surgical, radiotherapeutic or conservative.

Proptosis associated with acute inflammatory signs may indicate the possibility of orbital cellulitis, or the rare complication of cavernous sinus thrombosis.

PRACTICAL POINTS

● Stroke patients frequently lose all or part of the half field of each eye owing to involvement of the visual pathway. This is homonymous hemianopia, for which there is no available treatment.

● Transient visual loss is sometimes an indication of embolic cerebral disease. Clinical ausculation and angiography of the carotid are carried out where this condition is suspected.

● Aneurysms of the circle of Willis may produce compression of the lower visual pathway, pain in the region of the eye, or retinal haemorrhages leading to vitreous haemorrhage and sudden loss of vision.

● Cranial arteritis can lead to ischaemic papillopathy, with sudden complete blindness in the eye. The fellow eye can become affected very quickly, and an emergency estimation of the ESR is essential. Systemic steroids should be given immediately.

● Intracranial space-occupying lesions of the two types are associated with ocular effects: lower visual pathway compression and intracerebral lesions. If either is suspected, investigation is mandatory.
   Brain stem tumours can cause diplopia or, by interfering with cerebrospinal fluid circulation, papilloedema.

● In multiple sclerosis, there may be acute or progressive visual loss, as well as paralysis of the eye muscles and pupillary anomalies.

● In cases of loss of vision with no discernible pathology any of the following may be the cause: amblyopia, hysteria or malingering.

● Myasthenia gravis may cause ptosis or diplopia. It requires lifelong treatment with parasympathomimetic therapy. Thymectomy is appropriate in a few cases.

● Orbital disease may affect the optic or cranial nerves and produce proptosis. CT scans are an invaluable aid to diagnosis of orbital lesions.

25   Other specialties and ophthalmology

The interrelationships of ophthalmology with many of the subspecialties of medicine and surgery are reviewed and emphasis is again on the commonly occurring conditions. As an example, let us take dermatology. One condition discussed is rosacea, which may prompt a referral from an ophthalmologist to a skin specialist, or vice versa. The use of chloroquine for lupus erythematosus suggests to a dermatologist that an eye examination would be important. These interrelationships therefore cover both diagnosis and treatment, extending both to treatment for what might be an associated eye disorder and to any ocular side-effects of medication used in the specialty concerned.

PAEDIATRICS

The role of ophthalmology in paediatrics is examined under the following categories:

- The neonatal and early infantile period
- The premature infant
- The pre-school child
- Schoolchildren.

The neonatal and early infantile period

Shortly after birth all neonates should have their eyes routinely inspected to exclude obvious birth injuries, bruising of the eyelids, etc. Later, during this period, a more formal examination should take place, with particular reference given to the following conditions:

- Congenital abnormalities
- A red eye
- Discharge and sticky eyes
- Eye movements and squint
- The development of vision
- Congenital blindness
- Colour of the eyes.

Congenital abnormalities The shape and position of the eyelids should be noted. The eye itself may show a definite abnormality in the shape, size or colour of the pupils. The pupil reactions are often very slow, perhaps on account of the delay (up to three weeks postnatally) in myelination of the optic nerve. A poor or absent red reflex may indicate an anomaly of the media such as congenital cataract. The appearance of the eyes may give the first indication of Down's syndrome with its characteristic obliquity of the palpebral fissures.

A red eye in the neonatal or early infantile period (the classical 'ophthalmia neonatorum') is not very common. If it does occur, it is important to take a particular note of it as it may signify conjunctivitis with impending or actual corneal ulceration. Intensive local antibiotic treatment is given after cultures have been taken. Nowadays, the gonococcus (the classical cause of this condition) is rare. Chlamydial infection is said to be much more common. Prophylaxis of conjunctivitis by the routine instillation of chemotherapeutic drops at birth is important.

Discharge and sticky eyes Discharge from the eyes, without a particular inflammation, may simply be due to mild conjunctivitis or to a congenital lacrimal obstruction. In these latter cases in later infancy, copious pus may be expressed back into the conjunctival sac by pressure over the tear sac region. Usually the globe itself is not inflamed but if it is, a much more serious view of the situation is taken (see above).

After the neonatal period, a persistently sticky eye with or without watering again suggests lacrimal obstruction (see page 138). Much less commonly a micro-organism of a specific type (chlamydia, see above) may lead to chronic conjunctivitis.

The continuation of signs of congenital lacrimal obstruction in spite of expression of the tear sac, is an indication to consider probing of the nasolacrimal duct.

Eye movements and squint Until the neonate is about six weeks old, eye movements are uncoordinated. Eye fixation is unsteady and nystagmus-type movements may be seen. Variable and sometimes marked squints may be present, intermittently. By about six weeks of age, coordinated binocular fixation should begin as the eyes are kept open more and more of the time. Later in infancy, squint is often suspected when a very flat nose bridge with epicanthic folds is present.

The three important, basic strabismus examinations (inspection of the corneal reflections, the cover test and the ocular movements) have already been noted (see page 183) but it is worth restating that a suspicion or history of squint should prompt immediate referral, especially if a true squint is unquestionably present. Any delay may make amblyopia more difficult to treat, or postpone the diagnosis of a serious condition jeopardizing the sight of the squinting eye, as for example cataract, macular disease or even a retinal tumour (retinoblastoma).

Examination of the eye movements may show nystagmus. Persistence after the age of six weeks may indicate severe visual dysfunction, and in this connection the possibility of albinism should be raised.

The development of vision As noted above, shortly after six weeks of age an infant will begin to 'take notice' and the incoordination of the eyes becomes less frequent. The clinical tests of developing vision are simple at this period of life, consisting merely of observation as to the ability to follow a light and noting the pupil reactions. Later on, the facility to recognize familiar objects and parents' faces gives some indication of the standard of sight.

Congenital blindness Various forms of congenital blindness may be discovered in early infancy. Bilateral congenital cataract, perhaps caused by rubella, is one example. A parent will notice that the infant does not recognize him or her and seems unable to follow objects, except by sound. Often in such cases, nystagmus is present. One form in particular, known as Leber's optic atrophy, may present some diagnostic difficulty. This is because the infant's optic discs are normally pale, compared to their appearance later in life. True pallor representing optic atrophy in an infant may therefore be difficult to identify.

In all cases of doubt about an infant's vision, an examination under an anaesthetic with the pupils dilated is essential. In specialized units, electrodiagnostic tests (ERG, page 109; VER, page 249) may be available to confirm the absence or presence of a functioning retina and optic nerve.

The colour of the eyes usually develops during the course of the first year of life. The colour depends on the degree to which the front portion of the iris (the stroma) becomes pigmented. If this layer is poorly pigmented, the eye will be blue and, with increasing pigmentation, the eye shades pass through grey and green to hazel and brown. The back of the iris is a two-layered epithelium, heavily pigmented in all normal subjects. It is this layer and not the stroma that has the important light-excluding function. Defective pigmentation of the posterior iris epithelium is the direct cause of the photophobia experienced by the albino.

The premature infant

Prematurity has several important implications as far as the ophthalmologist is concerned. In particular, the excessive use of oxygen as a life-preserving measure in very low birthweight premature infants is known to be associated with the development of the condition of retrolental fibroplasia. While oxygen has been firmly implicated in the pathogenesis of this condition, there seems to be some kind of recrudescence of it in spite of the most careful monitoring of oxygen administration to neonates. The precise cause has not yet been elucidated, but in a clear and fully developed version of the condition, the high oxygen tension suppresses peripheral vas-

cular development of the retina. When the oxygen tension is reduced, an unbridled proliferation of vessels occurs, followed by fibrosis and shrinkage which leads to a total retinal detachment and a mass of scar tissue behind the lens in a completely blind eye. Incomplete forms of the condition exist and it may well be that another condition more frequently encountered in premature infants is a very mild version of it, that is, the association of some degree of myopia with prematurity. The myopia is of a different variety to that which affects adolescents later in life.

The pre-school child

The main condition to be considered in the pre-school child is concomitant strabismus (see Chapter 19), particularly the convergent variety. The critical period of onset is between two years and four years of age, although many strabismus cases may arise before this time and some are present at birth. Parents may put off seeking advice but there is often a fairly well defined start to the condition.

Particular attention should be paid to the history of squint coming on after measles or whooping cough or another debilitating illness. In all cases, a family history should be sought.

During this period of life a routine screening for both squint and defective vision can profitably be undertaken in child welfare clinics by family practitioners, by their nurses, or by orthoptists examining infants before entering school. Small angles of strabismus as well as defects of sight, perhaps of one eye only, may be detected early, before the parents have noticed anything amiss. This clearly makes earlier and therefore more successful treatment possible.

Special methods of testing vision are often necessary (Figures 25.1 and 25.2).

Schoolchildren

The ophthalmic problems of schoolchildren fall into three groups:

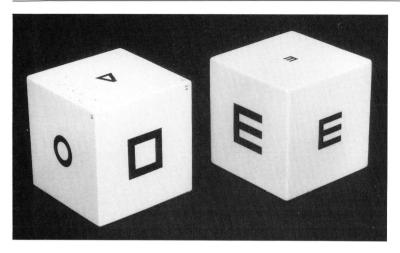

Figure 25.1 Methods of assessing visual acuity in children and, incidentally, in illiterates. The subject is asked to match the shape at the side of the cube, or the E, presented by the examiner at the appropriate distance (6 m).

- Simple visual difficulties (myopia, for example) that may be noticed by the child or parent, or both

- Reading problems

- Headaches.

Myopia usually occurs about the age of ten years, but may occasionally appear at younger ages, or even congenitally. Once discovered, periodic reassessment, perhaps twice a year, is advisable as it increases in degree throughout adolescence.

Reading problems Nowadays, reading problems are treated as part of an intricate and complex neuropsychological field of investigation. In all cases considered as dyslexia, a

routine eye examination, including refraction and orthoptic testing, is mandatory. As far as optical problems are concerned, significant astigmatism and moderate to high degrees of hypermetropia warrant the immediate wearing of spectacles. Low degrees of hypermetropia are commonly found, and are in fact the norm in the five to ten age group, but it is extremely unlikely to be beyond the capacity of children to overcome the condition by their own superabundant accommodative power. Spectacles successfully given to children for low hypermetropia may simply work as a placebo.

There is no real evidence that the monocularity of a child with a manifest unilateral squint is any impediment to the usual range of visual activity, including reading. On the other hand, the child who is binocular most of the time but has a latent squint may have difficulty in controlling it when

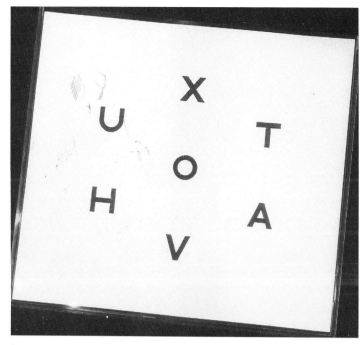

a

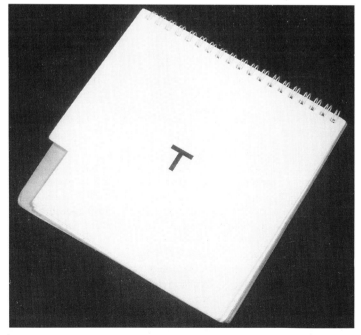

b

Figure 25.2 The Sheridan-Gardiner test: (*a*) the child holds the card and points to a letter which matches the one shown by the examiner 6 m away, then turns the flip-over (*b*), which has letters of progressively decreasing size.

reading, and blurring or inaccuracy of recognition may result. Convergence weakness is another cause of difficulty with reading, and orthoptic exercises may help.

Headaches may result both from simple refractive errors and from muscular imbalances similar to those producing eyestrain. Migraine and psychological causes are of course not infrequent in children, but it should never be forgotten that headache may be an important indication of general neurological disease (see page 227).

RHEUMATOLOGY

Not only are there direct association of eye disease with rheumatic conditions, but important iatrogenic complications may affect the eyes.

The most important condition is rheumatoid arthritis.

Rheumatoid arthritis

The condition exemplifies autoimmune disorders, and the eye may be involved in several

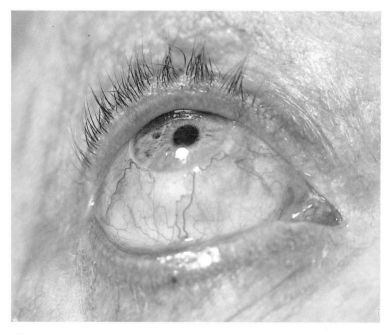

Figure 25.3 Scleromalacia perforans.

ways; Sjögren's syndrome (keratoconjunctivitis sicca) is frequently seen in patients with rheumatoid arthritis. The keratitis, in which epithelial filaments half-detach themselves from the corneal epithelium, produces irritable photophobic red eyes. The Schirmer test shows a virtual absence of tear production and this appears to be due to destruction of the lacrimal gland. The dye Rose-Bengal stains defective epithelium of both cornea and conjunctiva. Artificial tears should be given frequently. There are many varieties: normal saline, Ringer-Locke solution, methylcellulose and its close chemical relatives, as well as drops containing polyvinyl alcohol. Sealing of the lacrimal puncta temporarily with gelatin rods or permanently by cautery is sometimes helpful.

Other ocular problems in rheumatoids include scleritis/episcleritis and a curious 'cold' necrosis of the sclera, which progressively thins and produces bluish bulges; this is called scleroma lacia perforans. The colour is due to the unusual visibility of the underlying uvea (Figure 25.3).

The infantile form of rheumatoid arthritis (Still's disease) (Figure 25.4) is particularly liable to be accompanied by a severe anterior uveitis and to be complicated by cataract.

Some of the commonest eye problems arising in these patients are from the treatment. Prolonged systemic steroids may produce cataract and, rarely, glaucoma. Chloroquine or other antimalarial drugs give rise to a keratopathy which can cause the patient to see haloes round lights; of more importance is the retinal damage it may inflict. There is no means of predicting which patient will develop the problem, but to a certain extent the likelihood of occurrence is dose related. There is a need for close monitoring of the visual fields and fundus appearance, perhaps

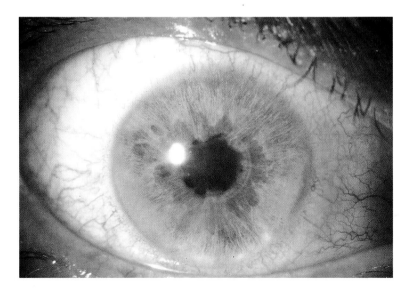

Figure 25.4 Old iridocyclitis in a case of Still's disease. Commencing calcification of the cornea can just be seen (band-shaped degeneration).

combined with electrodiagnostic tests of retinal function.

The important and frequent associations of ankylosing spondylitis with iritis deserves special mention, and is discussed in further detail in Chapter 9. Iritis is not common in rheumatoid arthritis.

Many of the autoimmune diseases may include polyarthritis among their manifestions and therefore come into the clinical field of the rheumatologist. Ocular involvements, similar to those in rheumatoid arthritis, may be found.

In addition, an arteritis (for example, poly-arteritis nodosa) may occur. Retinal and optic nerve vessel obstruction can result. Microinfarction of the retinal nerve fibre layer produces cytoid bodies typically seen in systemic lupus erythematosus. The arteritis of polymyalgia rheumatica can have similar occlusive effects on large or small retinal vessels.

Mention should also be made of Reiter's disease in which a polyarthritis may be present in association with urethritis and ocular inflammation, either keratitis or iritis.

EAR, NOSE AND THROAT

The following conditions and areas are discussed:

● Sinusitis

● Nasal congestion

● Trauma

● Tumours and mucocoeles

● Neuro-otology

● Orbital cellulitis.

Sinusitis

The proximity of the paranasal sinuses to the orbit has obvious implications. Pain due to sinus inflammation may be referred to the eye and acute ethmoiditis enters the differential diagnosis of acute inflammatory swellings at or near to the inner canthus.

Nasal congestion

Nasal congestion or other structural changes may obstruct the nasolacrimal duct. Some allergic conditions affect the nasal mucosa; for example, hay fever may similarly involve the conjunctiva. Itching and watering of the eyes are often features in such conditions.

Trauma

Trauma to the orbital bones may involve the rhinologist and the ophthalmologist, as well as the dentist and maxillofacial surgeon. Particular mention should be made of the blow-out fracture of the floor of the orbit (see page 173). Injury to the bridge of the nose can subsequently present problems in the wearing of spectacles.

Tumours and mucocoeles

Tumours and mucocoeles of the sinuses may encroach upon the orbit, thus displacing the eye forwards, laterally or medially (Figure 25.5). One of the earliest symptoms may be diplopia. Radical treatment of the lesions by surgery or radiotherapy can have serious ocular complications. Great care is exercised by the ENT surgeon to avoid disturbing the pulley of the superior oblique muscle, the trochlea, in procedures involving the frontal sinus.

When radiotherapy is used, it is often impossible to shield the eye adequately, the vision and health of which, if not already affected by the primary condition itself, are deliberately compromised. Such irradiated eyes become very inflamed with marked corneal epithelial disturbance and dryness (xerosis) of the conjunctiva. Lubrication, steroid and antibiotic drops should all be tried under an ophthalmologist's supervision.

Neuro-otology

The otologist is frequently active in the region of the facial nerve. Temporary or permanent interference with facial nerve function may lead to difficulty with closure of the lids, which may require tarsorrhaphy.

The science of neuro-otology revolves in part around the differential diagnosis of spontaneous and provoked nystagmus.

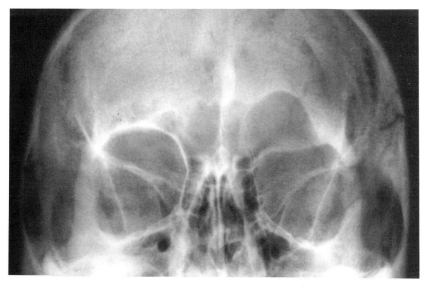

Figure 25.5 Mucocoele of the left frontal sinus. The x-ray shows the depression of the left orbital roof which this has produced.

VIth nerve involvement in petrous disease and loss of the corneal reflex in cerebellopontine angle tumours (deafness often being a presenting symptom) are other points of overlap between the two specialities.

Orbital cellulitis

The condition is characterized by painful swelling of the lids, chemosis (oedema of the conjunctiva), proptosis, and perhaps some interference with ocular movement (Figure 25.6). Infection of the sinuses is the most frequent cause.

Local and systemic chemotherapy for the ophthalmic condition is given in addition to measures directed to the underlying cause. Occasionally surgical evacuation of accumulations of pus is required.

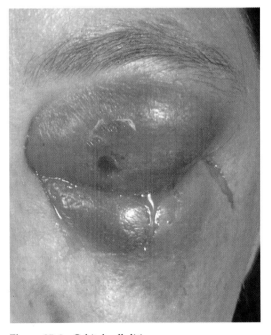

Figure 25.6   Orbital cellulitis.

DERMATOLOGY

It is hardly surprising that the epithelial surface of the conjunctiva and cornea should be disturbed in conditions affecting the epithelial surface of the skin; and the eyelids themselves are skin-covered. The interrelationship of skin and eye disease is enormous, but particular conditions stand out: blepharitis and atopic eczema.

Blepharitis

The common variety of blepharitis is often associated with seborrhoea. Less commonly, blepharitis is found in rosacea, an important condition in ophthalmology because of the associated keratitis which may occur. This usually takes the form of a superficial vascularized infiltration at the limbus (the corneoscleral junction), starting at the lower part of the cornea. More severe patches of inflammation can occur with ulceration and thinning and even perforation. Scleritis and episcleritis also occur in rosacea (Figures 25.7–25.9).

All forms of blepharitis may be associated with blocking of the meibomian glands and chalazia are common.

Rosaceal keratitis is responsive to topical steroid treatment.

Atopic eczema

In atopic eczema, typical involvement of the skin of the lids is found but in addition an epithelial keratopathy is seen, the patient suffering extreme photophobia and watering (Figure 25.10).

Eczematous lesions of the eyelids are very common manifestations of local or general allergic reactions.

Psoriasis

Psoriasis may be complicated by arthritis as well as by iritis. The treatment of psoriasis with

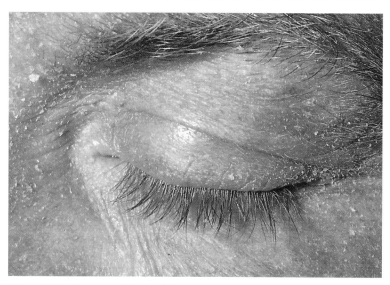

Figure 25.7 Rosacea of the eyelids.

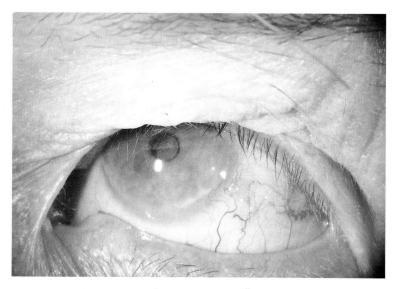

Figure 25.8 Old keratitis of the lower cornea in rosacea.

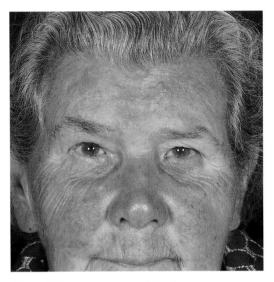

Figure 25.9   Acne rosacea of the face.

certain forms of ultraviolet radiation (PUVA) may call for supervision and protection of the eyes.

Vesicular lesions

Vesicular lesions of the skin have extremely important ocular associations. The two most important are herpes simplex (Figure 25.11) and herpes zoster (see also Chapter 8).

The rare bullous eruptions, erythema multiforme (Stevens-Johnson syndrome), pemphigus and dermatitis herpetiformis, may affect the conjunctiva with scarring lesions, sealing the inner lid surface to the globe (symblepharon) impairing ocular movement and possibly

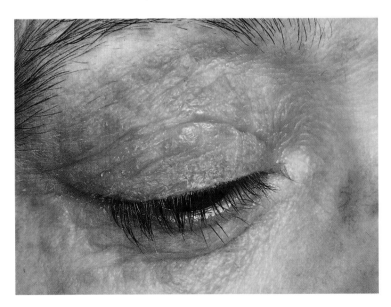

Figure 25.10   Atopic eczema of the eyelids. Such patients have an increased susceptibility to cataract and to keratoconus as well as to chronic corneal inflammation.

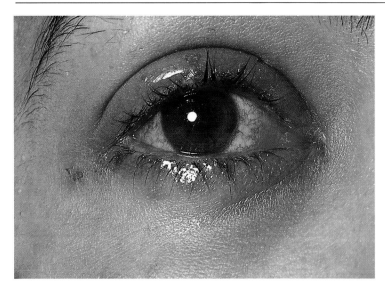

Figure 25.11   Viral conjuctivitis due to herpes simplex, which also affects the surrounding skin.

obstructing tear production. A milder form affects the eye and mucosae, and is known as benign mucous membrane pemphigoid. Orogenital ulceration occurs in Behçet's syndrome, an important if rare aetiology of uveitis and retinal arteritis.

Treatment of many of these conditions is by combined chemotherapy, steroids, lubrication of the eyes and mechanical separation of inflamed surfaces to prevent symblepharon.

Neoplasms

All manner of cutaneous tumours (see Chapter 17) may affect the skin of the eyelids. The vascular malformations such as strawberry marks may require cosmetic surgery, cryotherapy or photocoagulation.

The malignancies present special problems for the eye surgeon if radical extirpation means loss of the lids' protective function. Complex plastic reconstruction may be needed if it is felt that radiotherapy cannot adequately deal with the problem, or has failed. Lesions near the inner canthus are particularly beset with problems relating to tear drainage, whichever type of treatment is adopted.

GENERAL ANAESTHESIA

It is now recognized that general anaesthetics for any surgical procedure may be accompanied by an inadvertent exposure of the eyes. If there is the slightest suggestion of inadequate closure of the eyelids during a general surgical procedure, the lids should be taped closed until the patient has recovered from the anaesthetic.

If any recent ophthalmic operation has taken place, then all possible pressure on the eye by the hand or anaesthetic mask must be avoided. A plastic protective shield should cover the eye.

Most anaesthetists accept that in certain circumstances the use of the relaxant succinylcholine may lead to technical difficulties with intraocular surgery because of the contracture, often prolonged, of the extraocular muscles it produces. Many anaesthetists avoid its use altogether in eye work. It is especially to be eschewed if anaesthesia is to be given for repair of a penetrating eye injury.

The production of a 'relaxed' eye for the ophthalmic surgeon during intraocular surgery is part of modern anaesthetic skills which include general hypotension and reduction of the P_{CO_2} to decrease ocular vascularity, especially in the choroid.

A sign to both cataract surgeon and anaesthetist that excellent conditions have been produced is the spontaneous entry of an air bubble into the anterior chamber when the eye is opened. The most difficult circumstances for cataract surgery occur when the iris is so pushed forward that the anterior chamber is nonexistent and will not retain fluid or air when an attempt is made to introduce them. Surgical manipulation, both the removal of the cataract and the introduction of an intraocular lens, become hazardous in these conditions. Unfortunately this last situation cannot always be avoided by even the most refined anaesthetic techniques.

Pulling on the muscles during eye surgery, particularly during surgery to the muscles themselves, may lead to slowing of the heart-rate, but this is more of a problem of physiological interest rather than dire in its consequences.

The 'anaesthetic eye' is the term used to describe any red eye appearing in the immediate period after anaesthesia for any general surgical procedure. Its usual cause is an abrasion of the cornea because inadequate lid coverage has been allowed to occur during the anaesthesia. Occasionally such a red eye turns out to have acute glaucoma, due perhaps to a combination of emotion, atropine type drugs and an anatomical predisposition of the patient. Therefore, in all cases of 'anaesthetic eye', an ophthalmological opinion should be sought from the outset.

The anaesthetist is of course the ultimate arbiter as to the overall fitness for a general anaesthetic of a patient about to undergo eye surgery. If a general anaesthetic is undesirable, perfectly acceptable methods of local anaesthesia are available for ophthalmic surgery. These include local anaesthetic eyedrops such as cocaine or amethocaine and injections of lignocaine or bupivacaine, perhaps with very dilute adrenaline given into the retrobulbar space. These are combined with further infiltration of the eyelids, the muscle insertions and the upper branches of the facial nerve. Paralysis of the orbicularis oculi so induced prevents the patient squeezing his eye during surgery.

The attendance of an anaesthetist to give intravenous sedation may be helpful, even if preoperative sedation has already been given. A common routine is to give drugs of the benzodiazepine type, intravenously, in an age and weight related dosage.

ENDOCRINOLOGY

Dysthyroid eye disease—ophthalmic Graves' disease

This combination of physical signs and symptoms is one of the most common and important relationships between a systemic disorder and ophthalmology. The general disorder is usually, but not invariably, some degree of hyperthyroidism. Hypothyroidism, myxoedema, has a different eye picture (see page 271). The complex of hyperthyroidism consists of the following signs and symptoms:

● Proptosis due to abnormal fluid infiltration of orbital contents

● Retraction of the upper lid due to overaction of the levator muscle

● Diplopia due to malfunction of the extrinsic ocular muscles

● Visual loss due to the effects either of corneal exposure or of pressure on the optic nerve

● Fluid accumulation in the lids and conjunctiva.

Not all of these signs are necessarily present in any particular case, but the various signs tend to occur in fairly characteristic groups that can be loosely related to the stage of the dysthyroid condition.

Varieties of dysthyroid eye disease In classical thyrotoxicosis, bilateral proptosis occurs. It is usually not severe, but may be asymmetrical or even unilateral, and it should be remembered that the commonest cause of unilateral proptosis is dysthyroid disease. The protrusion of the eye is often slowly progressive for a limited period and then remains stationary.

The staring expression of the patient is an early sign of the thyrotoxic proptosis, and this appearance is aggravated by the upper lid retraction. The latter is responsible for several of the eye signs of thyrotoxicosis to which eponymous names have become attached:

● Graefe's sign is lid lag; failure to follow the eyeball on down gaze

● Joffroi's sign is excessive retraction of the upper lid on looking upwards

● Infrequent blinking.

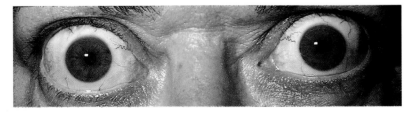

Figure 25.12 The typical stare of the patient with ophthalmic Graves' disease, thyrotoxicosis.

The fully developed picture of thyrotoxic bilateral upper lid retraction (Figure 25.12) is mimicked by very few conditions, perhaps the commonest of which is that produced by the discomfort of a poorly fitting contact lens. Very rarely, lid retraction is a manifestation of an upper brain stem disorder.

Diplopia is uncommon with the initial stages of thyrotoxicosis, as are the signs of fluid accumulation.

The clinical picture described above may be only partially abolished by medical or surgical control of the hyperthyroid state. The lid retraction may be reduced with some reduction of the stare but the proptosis often remains. In some cases the eye signs actually appear for the first time only after thyrotoxicosis has been controlled. This is particularly distressing for the patient who feels greatly improved in general health and has to face an unpleasant cosmetic problem.

In these circumstances, the condition may have rather different features and is sometimes referred to as thyrotropic exophthalmos, where it is believed that the reduction in the excess of circulating thyroid hormone allows the untrammelled effect of excessive pituitary thyrotropic hormone.

Thyrotropic exophthalmos, in its extreme form (Figure 25.13), may give rise to considerable anxiety for the continued health of the eyes. The condition may occur not only following the treatment of thyrotoxicosis but even in a person who has always been and continues to be an apparently euthyroid patient.

Proptosis occurs, which is much more severe and may in rare cases be rapidly progressive — 'malignant exophthalmos'.

Swelling of the lids and chemosis, conjunctival oedema, are common.

The extremes of dysthyroid eye diseases are at two ends of a spectrum. At one end there is hyperthyroidism with some proptosis and lid retraction but without much in the way of fluid accumulation in the lids and showing little interference with ocular movement. At the other end of the range we have a picture of severe proptosis, ocular muscle imbalance and swollen and congested conjunctivae and eyelids with or without hyperthyroidism. Between these two extremes, many mixed presentations occur.

Ocular exposure and its management

In proptosis the lids, like the conjunctiva, may be very fluid-laden, and may not completely

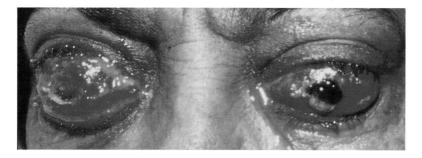

Figure 25.13   Severe so-called thyrotropic eye disease. The eyes are proptosed but in addition there is gross swelling of the lids and conjunctiva.

cover the cornea on attempted closure of the eyes. In milder degrees, some punctate staining with fluorescein of the lower cornea occurs, but this may proceed to abrasion and ulceration. In the most severe cases, perforation of the cornea can occur if measures are not taken to protect it.

If exposure is mild, lubricant drops such as hypromellose should always be given. Assuming that the lid retraction is due to excessive sympathetic stimulation of the involuntary part of the levator, guanethidine 5 per cent drops may have some effect. Some patients cannot tolerate these drops for long, as the eye becomes red and irritable.

Early tarsorrhaphy can be helpful from a cosmetic point of view and is advisable in more severe cases. Lateral tarsorrhaphy may be adequate. Temporary central tarsorrhaphy is mandatory if the cornea is ulcerated and fails to heal with conventional methods.

In extreme instances, and especially if it is felt that the sight is threatened not only by corneal ulceration but also by mechanical effects on the optic nerve in the orbit, orbital decompression is undertaken. This can be directed upwards by unroofing the orbit, laterally into the temporal fossa, or inwards and downwards into the sinuses.

Double vision due to dysthyroid disease

Interference with the action of the extraocular muscles may occur. This is partly due to mechanical inefficiency on account of the abnormally forward position of the globe, but the muscles themselves are abnormal. They may possibly be involved in a general dysthyroid myopathy but they are also directly infiltrated, perhaps with the same mucin laden fluid that fills the orbit. Certainly CT scanning of the orbits often shows clearly that the muscles are in fact enlarged (Figure 25.14). Indeed, if the patient is euthyroid, this particular diagnostic finding may be the sole indication of dysthyroid disease as the cause of proptosis, whether unilateral or bilateral. Some of the more recherché immunological tests also

seem to give evidence of the dysthyroid nature of certain cases of proptosis when there is no other evidence of disturbed thyroid function. In fact, the picture of ophthalmic Graves' disease is believed to be due to the reaction of the receptors on the muscles to antibody to thyroid stimulating hormone.

Clinically, vertical diplopia is most frequent and is often due to tethering of the inferior rectus muscle on one or both sides. In such cases, if prismatic spectacles do not help, controlled surgical recession may be required. It is usually best, if at all possible, to delay surgery until orthoptic examinations reveal that the condition is no longer progressive. Until then, covering one eye (occlusion) may be the only way to avoid double vision. Even if the condition is still progressive, surgery may sometimes be necessary.

The tethering of the inferior rectus is incidentally responsible for an interesting physical sign; the ocular pressure may rise significantly when the eye looks upwards or attempts to do so.

The place of systemic therapy

Systemic medical therapy specifically for dysthyroid eye disease is problematical. When given for thyrotoxicosis, the eye signs may resolve at least to some extent when the toxic element is brought under control, medically or surgically. As noted above, however, the opposite may occur and the eye signs may recur or indeed appear for the first time.

Non-surgical treatment for very severe dysthyroid proptosis is controversial but, in a proportion of patients, high doses of systemic steroids or steroid injections into the orbit are helpful. Radiotherapy to the orbit or the pituitary, or both, has also been tried. A presumed autoimmune element in the aetiology has prompted the use of immunosuppressive drugs such as azathioprine. Some success has also been claimed for plasmapheresis as a means of removing immune complexes; the technique may be employed alone or in combination with steroid therapy.

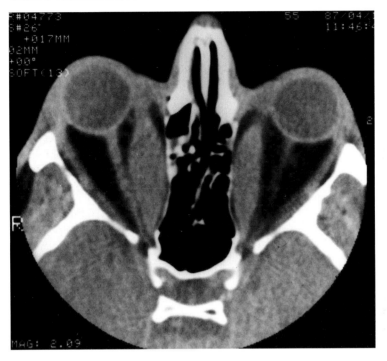

Figure 25.14   A CT scan of the orbit of the patient with
severe dysthyroid eye disease. Note the enormous
enlargement of the medial rectus muscle.

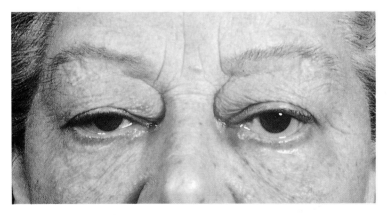

Figure 25.15   Myxoedema.

The marked oedema of the lids and conjunctiva sometimes responds to diuretics. Sleeping with the bedhead elevated may also help.

Myxoedema

The classical picture of hypothyroidism is typically marked by oedema of the lower lids and if hair loss is a feature, thinning of the outer third of the eyebrows (Figure 25.15).

Watering of the eyes is also a feature of myxoedema, but is experienced in other forms of dysthyroid disease for reasons which are not apparent.

Pituitary dysfunction

The condition may introduce important inter-relationships between endocrinology and ophthalmology. If hypophyseal swelling involves the optic chiasma, the vision and visual field of one or both eyes may be affected and the condition may present initially as an eye problem.

The classical bitemporal field loss of chiasmal compression, in the early stages frequently only to a red object, is less often found than an asymmetrical defect where the vision of one eye is significantly worse. Pallor of the disc of the affected eye parallels the degree of compression of the optic nerve.

Serial assessment by the ophthalmologist may show progressive field loss, indicating expansion of the lesion, or recovery of some field following surgical relief of the compression.

Similar monitoring of the visual fields is required during treatment with bromocriptine for infertility, as well as during pregnancy in patients with prolactinomas, as pituitary enlargement may occur.

The differential diagnosis of chiasmal compression by a pituitary swelling from other causes is discussed elsewhere (see Chapter 24), but the endocrine features which are suggestive include amenorrhoea in women and loss of facial hair in men, as well as a primary loss of sexual activity.

VENEREOLOGY

The ocular complications of syphilis are rare these days, whether the interstitial keratitis of congenital syphilis, the iritis of secondary syphilis, or the tabetic optic atrophy and Argyll Robertson pupils of neurosyphilis.

Even gonorrhoea is no longer the ocular scourge it was, owing to rapidly effective treatment. It is very uncommon to find ophthalmia neonatorum in modern obstetric practice and it is even rarer to encounter gonococcal uveitis in the adult.

Many recalcitrant causes of urethral discharge are known to be associated with ocular inflammation. Non-specific urethritis is sometimes accompanied by iritis and may occur with Reiter's syndrome. Chlamydial urethritis and cervicitis may be accompanied by a chronic conjunctivitis and corneal infiltration. Herpes simplex of the genitalia is mostly due to a strain of virus different to that which causes keratitis. Behçet's syndrome, in which genital ulceration features, has already been discussed (see page 265).

A lead in the diagnosis of AIDS is occasionally given by the ophthalmologist, who may find cytoid bodies (cotton wool spots) in the retina; anterior segment infection may be unexpected, prolonged or resistant to treatment. AIDS sufferers are prone to infection with toxoplasmosis and cytomegalic inclusion virus, both of which may seriously involve the retina, the latter infection often leading to retinal detachment. Conjunctival involvement by Kaposi's sarcoma also occurs.

TROPICAL DISEASES

Leprosy

In its lepromatous form inflammation of the anterior segment of the eye presents as conjunctivitis episcleritis, keratitis or as iridocyclitis. Cataract is a frequent complication (Figure 25.16).

The neural (tuberculoid) form may involve the Vth and VIIth cranial nerve, with failure of ocular protection caused by the inability of the lids to close over an anaesthetic cornea.

The acid-fast mycobacterium, Hansen's bacillus, is responsive to treatment with dapsone.

The general therapy is backed up by the standard specific measures for the particular ophthalmic problem which presents.

Onchocerciasis

The ocular effects of onchocerciasis, which is endemic in West Africa, are due to the dead microfilaria of the nematode worm, onchocerca volvulus. They include a severe keratitis and uveitis in the anterior segment, with choroidal sclerosis and optic atrophy in the fundus. Chemotherapy is directed against the microfilaria, for which diethylcarbamazine is the treatment, as well as against the adult worm, for which the therapy is suramin.

Trachoma

This chlamydial infection is reviewed more fully in Chapter 14. It is widespread not only in the

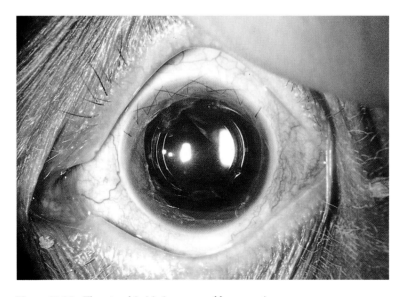

Figure 25.16 The atrophic iris in a case of leprosy. A posterior chamber implant has been inserted following cataract extraction. Its loop is visible where the iris is missing.

tropics, Africa, Asia and America, but also in Eastern Europe.

While in itself the involvement of the conjunctiva and the cornea by the chlamydial organism may not be severe, the effect of secondary infection and the scarring of the lid margins and cornea can have a devastating effect on vision.

As noted, trachoma remains perhaps the most important cause of blindness worldwide.

Cataract

Cataract is widespread in the tropics and its onset occurs at a generally earlier age than that at which senile cataracts occur in non-tropical climates. This has led to the postulation of sunlight as a causal factor.

A very substantial public health problem exists and is vigorously attacked by the 'eye-camp' organizations for performing cataract surgery, in India for example, on a huge scale. Perforce the techniques of cataract surgery are less sophisticated than in the conditions of developed societies. However, the excellent results are a tribute to the massive experience and skill of the surgeons who take part.

Nutritional disease

The principal nutritional disease affecting the eyes is xerophthalmia, due at least partly to vitamin A deficiency. The drying of the eye is associated with serious effects on both the conjunctiva and the cornea, which may ulcerate and lead to opacification and, in some cases, perforation with eventual blindness. There may be associated night blindness in other cases of vitamin A deficiency.

FURTHER ASSOCIATIONS WITH OPHTHALMOLOGY

While the associations are perhaps less apparent than in the foregoing conditions, common ground can be found between ophthalmology and the following specialties:

- Haematology
- Gastroenterology
- Chest medicine
- Nephrology.

Haematology

Every general clinical examination includes an inspection of the lower tarsal conjunctivae for pallor, which is found in anaemia.

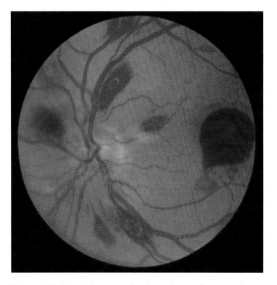

Figure 25.17   A haemorrhagic retinopathy seen in a case of leukaemia. Several of the haemorrhages have a characteristic white centre.

Cases of anaemia and the leukaemias may show retinal haemorrhage (Figure 25.17). In the leukaemias, some of these haemorrhages may have white centres. In pernicious anaemia there may be visual loss due to optic nerve dysfunction.

Treatment of leukaemias, as of other conditions of a neoplastic nature, may include immunosuppression and involve the use of systemic steroids and other agents. In such patients there is a marked increase in the liability to ocular infection by herpes simplex, particularly of the cornea and lids, and by cytomegalic inclusion virus, which may produce a particularly intractable form of retinitis.

Bleeding disorders rarely produce eye signs, but both retinal and subconjunctival haemorrhages do occasionally occur. Severe bleeding from a major body trauma or peptic ulceration, for example, may itself occasionally cause optic atrophy with permanent marked loss of vision.

Disturbances of the blood viscosity, as in some plasma protein anomalies and polycythaemia, may produce venous congestion in the retina.

Disorders of haemoglobin chemistry may show eye problems such as those found in sickle cell disease and trait. In sickle cell haemoglobin C disease, peripheral retinal vascular changes resembling periphlebitis are found with a marked tendency to vitreous haemorrhage and organization.

Gastroenterology

Gastroenterologists do not commonly come into contact with ophthalmology. Jaundice may cause yellowing of the conjunctivae. Chronic bowel inflammation is sometimes associated with episcleritis or iritis. Parasympatholytic drugs used in treatment may produce visual side-effects. Cases of hepatic disorder due to Wilson's disease (hepato-lenticular degeneration) may show a deposit in the corneal periphery, the Kayser-Fleischer brown ring (Figure 25.18). In its early stages the 'ring' is visible only on the slit-lamp, but it is pathognomonic of the condition.

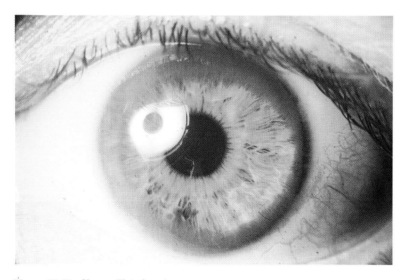

Figure 25.18   Kayser-Fleischer ring.

Liver disease may be one cause of vitamin A deficiency. As this vitamin is essential for the production of visual purple, the pigment of the rods, lack of it may lead to night blindness. Liver failure may also be associated with a bleeding tendency, manifesting itself in haemorrhages in the lids of the conjunctiva.

Chest medicine

The chest physician often asks the ophthalmologist to check the continuing visual function in patients treated with antituberculous therapy, particularly ethambutol because of its ocular toxicity.

Chest signs (radiological or otherwise) may be the first indication of sarcoidosis, for which the chest physician might seek an ophthalmologist's opinion. Findings suggesting the presence of sarcoidosis include evidence of active or past uveitis, particularly anterior uveitis; swelling of the lacrimal and parotid glands; and dryness of the eyes if there is some autoimmune suppression of lacrimal secretion. Occasionally there are granulomata present in the conjunctiva. Finally, some cases of sarcoidosis show retinal vasculitis.

Nephrology

Besides the retinal problems associated with high blood pressure (see pages 219–20), patients with renal failure may show corneal calcification. Any generalized oedema may involve the eyelids. Renal transplantation often requires anti-rejection therapy, which itself brings eye problems such as a steroid cataract.

PRACTICAL POINTS

● Rheumatoid arthritis may be associated with irritable photophobic red eyes owing to filamentary keratitis. This is caused by an absence of tears owing to destruction of the lacrimal gland. Artificial tears should be administered frequently.

● Infantile rheumatoid arthritis (Still's disease) is likely to be accompanied by uveitis and complicated by cataract.

● Acute ethmoiditis is part of the differential diagnosis of inflammatory swelling at the inner canthus.

● Itching and watering eyes are features of hay fever involving the nasal mucosa and conjunctiva.

● Orbital cellulitis, frequently due to infected sinuses, is treated by local or systemic chemotherapy. Occasionally evacuation of pus is necessary.

● Blepharitis is associated with seborrhoea, and sometimes rosacea. Severe inflammation in the latter condition can result in ulceration and thinning of the cornea.

● Vesicular lesions of the skin may have very serious implications for eyes. The most common lesions causing such problems are those produced by herpes simplex and herpes zoster. Rarely, bullous eruptions may affect the conjunctiva, sealing the inner lid to the globe.

● An 'anaesthetic' red eye should always be investigated by the ophthalmologist for corneal abrasion or glaucoma.

● Dysthyroid disease has some of the most obvious and well known ocular symptoms, including:
— Proptosis, perhaps with corneal exposure
— Retraction of the upper lid
— Diplopia.

● Early ocular exposure may be managed by eye drops. In severe cases, tarsorrhaphy may be necessary, or even orbital decompression.

● Hypothyroidism is typified by oedema of the lower lids and watering eyes.

● AIDS may sometimes be indicated by cotton wool spots in the retina or resistant anterior or posterior segment infection.

● Trachoma is the most important cause of blindness worldwide. It is widespread not only in the tropics, Africa, Asia and America, but also in Eastern Europe.

Select bibliography

General texts

DUANE, T.D., *Clinical ophthalmology* 5 vols (London: Harper & Row, 1979).

KANSKI, J.J., *Clinical ophthalmology* (London: Butterworths, 1984).

MILLER, S.J.H., *Clinical ophthalmology* (Bristol: Wright, 1987).

MILLER, S.J.H., *Parson's diseases of the eye* 17th edn (Edinburgh: Churchill Livingstone, 1984).

VAUGHAN, D. and ASBURY, T., *General ophthalmology* 11th edn (Los Altos: Lange Medical, 1986).

Cataract

SINSKEY, R.M. and BLASE, W.P., *Manual of cataract surgery* (New York: Churchill Livingstone, 1987).

Glaucoma

EPSTEIN, D.L. (ed), *Chandler and Grant's Glaucoma* 3rd edn (Philadelphia: Lea & Febiger, 1986).

Injuries

EAGLING, E.M. and ROPER-HALL, M.J., *Eye injuries: an illustrated guide* (London: Gower Medical, 1986).

Medical ophthalmology

DINNING, W.J., *Systemic inflammatory disease and the eye* (Bristol: John Wright, 1987).

ROSE, F.C., *Eye in general medicine* (London: Chapman & Hall, 1983).

Optics

DUKE-ELDER, S., *Practice of refraction* 9th edn (Edinburgh: Churchill Livingstone, 1978).

ELKINGTON, A.R. and FRANK, H., *Clinical optics* (Oxford: Blackwell Scientific, 1984).

Retinal detachment

SCHUTZ, J.S., *Retinal detachment surgery: strategy and tactics* (London: Chapman & Hall, 1984).

Strabismus

HARCOURT, B. and MEIN, J., *Diagnosis and management of ocular motility disorders* (Oxford: Blackwell Scientific, 1986).

Uveitis

KANSKI, J.J., *Uveitis: a colour manual of diagnosis and treatment* (London: Butterworths, 1987).

Index

Page numbers in *italic* refer to the illustrations